KEY QUESTIO

RADIOLOG

KEY QUESTIONS IN
RADIOLOGY

Paul Hulse
MRCP FRCR
Senior Registrar in Radiology
Department of Diagnostic Radiology
University of Manchester

Mark Callaway
MRCP
Registrar in Radiology
Department of Diagnostic Radiology
University of Manchester

Nigel Hoggard
MRCP
Registrar in Radiology
Department of Diagnostic Radiology
University of Manchester

Michael Roberts
BSc
Lecturer in Physics
University College Salford

βIOS
SCIENTIFIC
PUBLISHERS

©BIOS Scientific Publishers Limited 1996

First published 1996

A CIP catalogue record for this book is available from the British Library.

ISBN 1 85996 245 9

BIOS Scientific Publishers Limited,
9 Newtec Place, Magdalen Road, Oxford OX4 1RE, UK.
Tel: +44 (0)1865 726286, Fax: +44 (0)1865 246823.
World Wide Web home page: http://www.Bookshop.co.uk/BIOS/

DISTRIBUTORS

Australia and New Zealand
    DA Information Services
    648 Whitehorse Road, Mitcham
    Victoria 3132, Australia

India
    Viva Books Private Ltd
    4325/3 Ansari Road, Daryaganj
    New Dehli 110002

Singapore and South East Asia
    Toppan Company (S) PTE Ltd
    38 Liu Fang Road, Jurong
    Singapore 2262

USA and Canada
    BIOS Scientific Publishers
    PO Box 605
    Herndon VA 22070

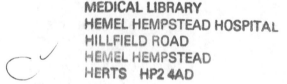
Typeset by Els Boonen, BIOS Scientific Publishers Ltd, Oxford, UK.
Printed by Redwood Books, Trowbridge, UK.

CONTENTS

ABBREVIATIONS

AICA	Anterior inferior cerebellar artery
ALARA	As low as reasonably achievable
AP	Antero-posterior
ARSAC	Administration of Radioactive Substances Advisory Committee
ASIS	Anterior superior iliac spine
AXR	Abdominal X-ray
BPD	Bi-parietal diameter
Bq	Becquerel
CBD	Common bile duct
CHD	Common hepatic duct
Co	Cobalt
CSF	Cerebrospinal fluid
CsI	Caesium iodide
CT	Computed tomography
D	Density
DMSA	Dimercaptosuccinic acid
DS	Observed frequency
DTPA	Diethylene triamine pentacetic acid
ERCP	Endoscopic retrograde cholangiopancreatogram
eV	Electronvolts
FFD	Focus-film distance
FFP	Fresh frozen plasma
G	Gauss
GFR	Glomerular filtration rate
GI	Gastrointestinal
h	Plancks constant
Hz	Hertz
I	Intensity
IA DSA	Intraarterial digital subtraction angiography
ICRP	International Committee on Radiation Protection
IM	Intramuscular
IRR	Ionizing Radiation Regulations
IUCD	Intrauterine contraceptive device
IVC	Inferior vena cava
IV DSA	Intravenous digital subtraction angiography
IVP	Intravenous pyelogram
IVU	Intravenous urogram
KUB	Kidneys, ureters and bladder
kV	Kilovolts

LAO	Left anterior oblique
LPO	Left posterior oblique
MAA	Microaggregated albumin
MAG 3	Mercaptoacetyltriglycine
MDP	Methylene disphosphonate
MeV	Megaelectronvolts
MR	Magnetic resonance
MRI	Magnetic resonance imaging
MTF	Modulation transfer function
NRPB	National Radiological Protection Board
OFD	Object-film distance
PA	Posterior-anterior
PE	Pulmonary embolus
PET	Positron emission tomography
PMT	Photomultiplier tube
POPUMET	Protection of persons undergoing medical examination or treatment
PRF	Pulse repetition frequency
PTFE	Polytetrafluoroethylene
QC	Quality control
RAO	Right anterior oblique
RBE	Relative biological effectiveness
RCR	Royal College of Radiologists
RF	Radiofrequency
s	Second
SMV	Submentovertical
SPTA	Spatial peak temporal average
STIR	Short term inversion recovery
Sv	Sieverts
T1	Longitudinal relaxation time
Tc	Technetium
Tc-99m	Metastable technetium
TE	Time to echo
TGC	Time gain compensator
TLD	Thermoluminescence dosimeter
TOF	Tracheo-oesophageal fistula
TR	Time to repeat
UBO	Unidentified bright object
UTI	Urinary tract infection
w/v	Weight by volume
Z	Acoustic impedence

PREFACE

This book is primarily for radiologists preparing for the Part 1 examination of the Royal College of Radiologists (Clinical Radiology) but will also be of value to those radiographers who are learning or revising for examinations. We have tried to adhere closely to the Part 1 syllabus issued by the college, which is admirably explicit, particularly in the physics section.

The questions are in the true/false format used in most British Postgraduate Medical examinations. Candidates score one mark for a correct response and have one mark deducted for an incorrect answer. No marks are given if the question is unanswered. Each examination has 20 physics, 20 anatomy and 20 techniques questions. An overall mark can be used to monitor progress with your revision, but highlighting weak areas of knowledge requiring attention is a much more useful exercise. Most of the questions are very straightforward and intended to test or illustrate a particular point. There are some more difficult ones to test the knowledge and examination skills of 'Gold Medal' students. The material has been largely drawn from the books listed in the bibliography (see page 114) but a reference is given if the answer is to be found elsewhere.

We are very grateful to Dr Jonathan Fields, of the Department of Diagnostic Radiology, University of Manchester, and to Dr Alan Hufton of the North West Regional Medical Physics Department, Christie Hospital, Manchester, who carefully reviewed the questions and made many helpful suggestions.

Good luck with your revision and the exam.

Paul Hulse
Mark Callaway
Nigel Hoggard
Michael Roberts

FOREWORD

All those undergoing specialist medical training have the daunting hurdles of examinations to pass to achieve their required professional credentials. Doctors in their first year of radiological training are no exception and have much new and varied knowledge to acquire - in physics, anatomy and techniques - in preparation for the Part 1 Fellowship examination of the Royal College of Radiologists. Like them or not - we all have to accept that multiple choice questions are established as a proven and widely applied method for assessing the knowledge of examination candidates. This book, I feel sure, will prove valuable in the preparation for this examination. The questions are grouped and presented in a style close to that of the actual examination, which is particularly useful, and candidates can use the book to provide 'mock' examination papers to assess their performance - before facing the real thing! With the true/false answers being provided, some with additional explanatory information, the book also serves to add to candidates' knowledge.

The authors are well aware of what a book such as this needs to offer to readers. The stimulus to prepare it developed while some were in the throes of preparing for the examination themselves. Collecting and verifying the questions and answers is a considerable task which the authors completed soon after putting this particular examination hurdle behind them; I applaud their enterprise and achievement.

Professor Judith E. Adams FRCP FRCR
Professor of Diagnostic Radiology, University of Manchester, and
Honorary Consultant Radiologist, Central Manchester Healthcare Trust

EXAMINATION ONE

Allow 2 hours for the completion of all 60 questions
Answers are on page 71

1.1   Regarding atomic structure

A K shell electrons are found in the atomic nucleus
B orbital electrons are bound by the nucleus and must be given energy to escape
C the K shell electron energy level for tungsten is the same as that for aluminium
D electron energy levels in an atom are equally spaced
E L shell electrons have less kinetic energy than M shell electrons

1.2   Concerning the interaction of X-rays with matter

A during elastic scattering partial absorption occurs
B Compton interactions occur with free electrons
C a Compton scattered photon can be emitted in any direction
D as X-ray photon energy increases there is less Compton scattering
E during pair production the incident photon must have energy of greater than 0.51 MeV

1.3   Regarding the electromagnetic spectrum

A the intensity of a beam of X-rays is measured in J/sec
B the energy of a photon of light increases with its frequency
C gamma rays are emitted as a result of interactions within the nucleus
D Plancks constant has the same units as frequency
E X-rays and gamma rays never display particle-like activity

1.4   Concerning IRR 85

A it is the responsibility of the employee to monitor and maintain the safety of equipment
B a controlled area is one in which doses are likely to exceed 30% of any dose limit for employees over 18 years of age
C dose limits are irrelevant when defining a supervised area
D controlled and supervised areas are defined in the 'systems of work'
E local rules allow non-classified persons to enter a controlled area

1.5 Regarding units

A the unit of exposure is joules per kilogram (J/kg)
B the unit of absorbed dose is the sievert
C 1 gray is equal to 1 joule per kilogram (J/kg)
D equivalent dose and effective dose are measured in the same units
E collective dose is measured in man sieverts

1.6 Film badges for personal monitoring

A consist of a single emulsion film mounted in a holder
B should be changed 6-monthly
C will usually indicate if the wearer has been in the primary beam
D may be calibrated using a radioactive source
E give information about the type and energy of radiation received

1.7 Tungsten is used as the filament in an X-ray tube because it

A has a high specific heat capacity
B has a high atomic number
C is ductile
D can be easily replaced
E gives a large thermionic emission

1.8 Geometric unsharpness in radiology

A is minimized by using the smallest possible focal spot
B is increased by increasing the focus-film distance (FFD)
C is increased by increasing the object-film distance (OFD)
D is minimized by using arrested inspiration
E is dependent on kV

1.9 Regarding X-ray film cassettes

A placing a wire mesh inside the cassette is used to test the film screen contact
B the film-screen combination is removed during 'daylight' processing
C just the film is removed during processing in the dark room
D contains a lead blocker which absorbs radiation during exposure
E may be used in any orientation

1.10 In computed tomography

A the window width controls range of CT numbers between white and black
B the CT number of a voxel increases with the attenuation of the X-ray beam
C mechanical misalignment causes ring artefacts
D data acquisition times are usually longer than for MRI
E the partial volume effect is increased with increased slice thickness

1.11 Regarding X-ray grids

A crossed grids are used when tube angulation is needed
B grid movement is synchronized with X-ray pulse production
C grid movement increases patient dose
D bucky (or grid) factor expresses the increased exposure required by the use of a grid
E focused grids are used to direct the primary beam towards the detector

1.12 Regarding image intensifiers

A image intensity increases with fluorescent screen thickness
B fluorescent screens consist of a single large crystal of CsI
C light photons emitted by the CsI screen are accelerated by potential difference between input and output phosphors
D the output screen is smaller than the input screen to give increased brightness
E electrodes between photocathode and output screen are used to focus electron beams

1.13 Concerning ultrasound

A refraction is governed by Snell's law
B the proportion of sound reflected is related to the relative densities at an interface
C acoustic impedance of air is greater than that of fat
D below a certain incident angle a large proportion of the beam is reflected towards the transducer
E increasing the frequency of a beam reduces its intensity at any given point in a patient

1.14 Regarding artefacts in ultrasound

A interference from multiple reflections can be of value

B acoustic enhancement in abdominal scanning can result in an image of the liver lying in the lung

C pelvic scanning with a full bladder uses acoustic shadowing

D aliasing is reduced by reducing the frequency of the transducer

E a tissue interface maybe misinterpreted because of reflection off the transducer

1.15 Concerning ultrasound transducers

A with a linear array, electronic focusing is achieved by triggering the inner elements prior to the outer ones

B a curvilinear array produces a sector shaped field

C reducing the sector angle increases the frame rate of a phased array

D beam steering is optimal with an annular array

E require a thin matching layer as well as the coupling oil or gel

1.16 The Larmor frequency in MRI

A is the frequency at which the protons spin on their axes

B is independent of the strength of the external magnetic field

C is directly proportional to the gyromagnetic ratio

D is in the microwave frequency band of the electromagnetic spectrum

E varies between patients

1.17 The longitudinal relaxation time (T1) in MRI

A is also called spin-spin relaxation time

B is the time taken for each magnetic moment to return to its original orientation

C is the time for the longitudinal magnetization to return to 63% of its original value

D is between 30 ms and 100 msec in biological tissue

E cannot be measured directly

1.18   **Regarding pulse sequences in MRI**

A   inversion recovery sequences provide good contrast in soft tissue
B   a saturation recovery sequence involves two 90° pulses separated by a short TR
C   in a spin-echo sequence, the signal is measured immediately after the 180° pulse
D   proton density images are produced by a spin-echo sequence with long TR and long TE
E   partial saturation sequences give T1 weighted images

1.19   **Regarding quality control (QC) of a gamma camera system**

A   QC need only be carried out weekly
B   measurement of energy resolution requires two distinct sources
C   sensitivity is measured using a point source
D   QC includes measurement of the speed of rotation of the camera head
E   QC includes a measurement of the residual activity of the camera head

1.20   **Tc-99m radiopharmaceuticals**

A   must be administered on the day of production
B   are generally chemically stable for only 4-8 hours after production
C   must be produced in aseptic conditions
D   are stored in 3 mm lead pots
E   are produced from radioactive, freeze-dried chemical 'kits'

1.21   **The following bones have a membranous ossification**

A   mandible
B   maxilla
C   squamous part of the occiput
D   hyoid
E   vomer

1.22   **The following structures pass through the superior orbital fissure**

A   ophthalmic veins
B   inferior oculomotor nerve
C   abducent nerve
D   maxillary nerve
E   optic nerve

1.23 The following branch directly from the external carotid artery

A inferior thyroid artery
B ophthalmic artery
C facial artery
D middle meningeal artery
E maxillary artery

1.24 Cerebrospinal fluid

A has a volume of around 200 ml
B has a re circulation of 8-10 x per 24 h
C is contained within the subarachnoid space
D has a higher protein concentration at the cephalic rather than caudal end
E contains immunoglobulins

1.25 A normal oesophagus

A receives blood from the inferior thyroid artery
B is indented at C6 by the post cricoid venous plexus
C receives only sympathetic supply from the oesophageal plexus
D has a 'B ring' that is visible on a normal barium swallow
E is about 40 cm in length

1.26 Concerning the diaphragm

A the right crus arises from L1,2,3 vertebral bodies
B the right hemidiaphragm is up to 2 cm higher than the left
C the left gastric artery and vagus nerve pass through at T10
D the right, but not left lateral arcuate ligament arches over quadratus lumborum muscle
E the left phrenic nerve passes through at T8

1.27 The spleen

A has a length of 12 cm
B has direct attachment to the stomach via the greater omentum
C is most likely to develop an accessory lobe inferiorly
D is suspended at its hilum by two ligaments
E has lymphatic drainage to the pre-aortic nodes

1.28 Regarding the normal duodenum

A it is completely retroperitoneal
B it has no mesentery along the 2nd part
C it is traversed anteriorly along the 3rd part by the inferior mesenteric artery
D the duodenal-jejunal flexure is supported by the ligament of Trietz
E the accessory duct of Santorini may open directly into it

1.29 The intrathoraic azygos vein

A arches over the root of the right lung
B originates in the abdomen
C receives blood from the oesophageal veins
D has a maximum diameter of 1 cm in an adult
E is decreased in size by a Valsalva manoeuvre

1.30 Concerning the mediastinum at the level of T3

A the left brachiocephalic vein is present
B the trachea is directly related to the brachiocephalic artery
C the phrenic nerve is anterior to the vagus
D the thoracic duct is posterior to the oesophagus
E both common carotid arteries are present

1.31 Regarding the thoracic great vessels

A the right subclavian artery passes posterior to the oesophagus in up to 1% of adults
B the left vertebral artery arises from the arch of the aorta in up to 5% of adults
C the arch of the aorta lies posterior to the thymus
D the arch of the aorta is connected to the pulmonary trunk by the ligamentum arteriosum
E the left common carotid artery arises from the brachocephalic artery in up to 10% of people

1.32 Concerning the lungs

A the oblique fissure lies in a line between the spine of the 3rd thoracic vertebra and the 6th costochondral junction
B a carinal angle of 60 degrees is normal
C the horizontal fissure is in a line between the 6th right costal cartilage and the oblique fissure
D the left hilum may normally be 2 cm above the right
E on full inspiration the right hemidiaphragm should reach the anterior end of the right 6th rib

1.33 The following bones lie in close apposition

A os peroneum: cuboid
B os trigonum: talus
C os tibiale externum: 5th metatarsal
D os supratalare: talus
E os intermetatarseum: 5th metatarsal

1.34 The lunate articulates with the following bones

A triquetral
B trapezoid
C capitate
D hamate
E scaphoid

1.35 Concerning the knee

A the ossification centre of the patella is present at birth
B the lateral collateral ligament is external to the capsule
C the posterior cruciate ligament passes from the anterior intercondylar region to the lateral aspect of the medial femoral condyle
D the patella has a larger medial articular surface
E the patella may normally be segmented

1.36 Concerning pelvimetry, the minimum normal values are

A AP inlet: 13 cm
B AP outlet: 12 cm
C transverse inlet: 11.5 cm
D interspinous: 9 cm
E femoral neck angle in adult: 160 degrees

1.37 **Concerning the embryology of the heart**

A the foramen ovale joins the right and left ventricle
B the ductus arteriosus joins the right pulmonary artery to the descend-
ing aorta
C the ductus venosus enters directly into the right atrium
D the left umbilical artery carries deoxygenated blood in the fetus
E the right umbilical artery is a branch of the common iliac artery

1.38 **The urinary bladder**

A contains transitional epithelium
B receives its blood supply from branches of the internal iliac artery
C receives innervation from L1 and L2
D is under inhibitory control of the corticospinal tract
E has a trigone limited by the interureteric ridge

1.39 **The thyroid gland**

A is at the level of C6
B drains blood to both the internal jugular and brachiocephalic vein
C is derived from the 3rd and 4th pharyngeal pouch
D may contain the parathyroid glands in its capsule
E the pyramidal lobe arises from the lateral lobe

1.40 **Concerning the ear**

A the medial end of the auditory tubes lies in the temporal bone
B the incus is in contact with the tympanic membrane
C the stapedius and tensor tympani are supplied by the facial nerve
D the glossopharyngeal nerve supplies the middle ear
E the cochlear duct contains endolymph

1.41 **Regarding oral cholecystography**

A a low kV is used for the control film
B modern contrast media are protein bound *in vivo*
C a total of 3 g of contrast media taken in divided doses is conventional
D an erect view is important
E the cystic duct and common ducts are seen in greater detail following
fatty meal stimulation

1.42 Concerning a T-tube cholangiogram

A fluoroscopy is required
B the T-tube should be clamped prior to the examination
C aspiration of bile is part of the procedure
D spasm of the sphincter of Oddi may mimic a common duct calculus
E the T-tube is withdrawn prior to removal of a calculus

1.43 Concerning myelography

A it should not be performed on the day following a lumbar puncture
B sedation is routinely required
C local anaesthesia is usually required
D no more than 1.5 g of iodine should be injected into the subarachnoid space
E patients should be observed in hospital for at least 12 hours after the procedure

1.44 Regarding lower limb venography

A it is of value in the demonstration of incompetent perforating veins
B it is of value in the investigation of venous ulceration
C it is contraindicated if the patient is anticoagulated
D the patient should be fasted prior to the procedure
E cellulitis is a contraindication

1.45 In phaeochromocytoma a hypertensive crisis maybe precipitated by

A hyoscine-n-butyl bromide
B glucagon
C metoclopramide
D phentolamine
E sodium diatrizoate

1.46 Concerning ionic iodinated contrast media

A pure sodium salts should be used for neuro-angiography
B pure methyl-glucamine (meglumine) salts are desirable for cardio-angiography
C sodium salts are more painful in arteries than meglumine salts
D meglumine salts are less irritant to veins than sodium salts
E may be used for myelography

1.47 Concerning gastrointestinal contrast media

A a concentration of 100% w/v barium sulphate is best used for a double contrast barium meal

B high density preparations (200-250% w/v) are used for barium enemas

C gastrografin is best used for a video swallow in a patient who has suffered a recent stroke

D the bladder may become opacified during a gastrografin swallow

E only single contrast studies are adequate with water soluble agents

1.48 The following are visible on a standard 20 degrees occipito-frontal skull radiograph

A crista galli

B odontoid peg

C mastoid process

D basi-occiput

E foramen rotundum

1.49 The patient position for the following radiographs is correct

A right posterior oblique for the left sacro-iliac joint

B left anterior oblique for the right upper ribs

C right anterior oblique for the left sternoclavicular joint

D right anterior oblique for a lateral view of the right scapula

E left anterior oblique for the left sided pars interarticularis of the lumbar spine

1.50 Concerning a ^{99m}Tc pertechnetate brain scan

A the radiopharmaceutical accumulates in normal choroid plexus

B the administered activity is about 350-500 MBq

C the radiopharmaceutical crosses the intact blood-brain barrier

D 500 mg of potassium perchlorate is required prior to injection of the radiopharmaceutical

E the scalp and underlying muscles are normally seen

1.51 Renal radionuclide studies maybe useful in the evaluation of

A renal failure
B renal trauma
C transitional cell carcinoma of the urinary tract
D vesico-ureteric reflux
E hypertension

1.52 Sialography is indicated

A for xerostomia
B for sialorrhoea
C in the presence of a known salivary calculus
D for bilateral parotid swelling
E for purulent discharge from the parotid (Stensens) duct

1.53 Regarding examination of the paediatric oesophagus

A dilute barium is required to demonstrate oesophageal atresia
B it is possible to assess the extent of an atretic segment on a chest radiograph
C during demonstration of a tracheo-oesophageal fistula (TOF) the table should be horizontal and the infant held horizontally, face down
D the oesophagus should be maximally distended with contrast in order to demonstrate a TOF
E the oesophagus should be maximally distended with barium in order to demonstrate vascular rings

1.54 Concerning preparation for a barium enema

A on the day of the examination, diabetics should defer oral hypoglycaemics until after the examination is finished
B a normal insulin regime should be taken by an insulin dependent diabetic on the day of the examination
C patients with renal impairment require special preparation
D picolax forms two active components when dissolved in water
E following the use of a cleansing water enema a delay is required before the examination

1.55 The following are true about patient preparation for CT scanning

A conventional barium studies should be performed before abdominal scanning is considered

B a 3 hour fast is required prior to an abdominal scan

C men should empty their bladders before pelvic scanning

D oral contrast media is needed when examining the pancreas

E smoking is forbidden for 24 hours before imaging of the mediastinum

1.56 Concerning magnetic resonance imaging

A on a T2 weighted brain scan the CSF appears white

B fat in the scalp is of low signal intensity on T1 and T2 weighted scans

C cortical bone gives a signal void from a 'proton density' spin-echo sequence

D intraperitoneal fat appears dark grey on a short term inversion recovery (STIR) sequence

E mascara may cause local susceptibility artefacts

1.57 Regarding pelvic ultrasound

A the external uterine os lies beneath the point at which the posterior wall of the bladder appears to change direction

B the width of the endometrium increases through the menstrual cycle

C the ovaries are less echogenic than the uterus

D visualization of the ovaries may be confirmed by seeing the ovarian vessels entering postero-medially

E after hysterectomy the levator ani muscle may be mistaken for an ovary

1.58 Regarding the umbilical vein on obstetric ultrasound

A it travels horizontally through the liver

B it joins the left branch of the portal vein

C when measuring abdominal circumference, it should be seen in its maximum possible extent

D the spine may cast an acoustic shadow over it

E it forms a cruciate arrangement with the two branches of the portal vein and the umbilical artery

1.59   Intravenous urography

A   is valuable for determining the presence of renal artery stenosis
B   should be performed following a bout of epididymo-orchitis
C   is essential in women with recurrent urinary tract infections
D   is contraindicated in all diabetics with renal impairment
E   should not be performed following a ^{123}I sodium iodide thyroid scan

1.60   Concerning retrograde pyelography

A   it is usually required because of inadequate IV urography
B   it is contraindicated if a ureteric neoplasm is suspected
C   it is preferable for the radiologist to catheterize the ureter
D   the tip of the catheter should initially lie in the renal pelvis
E   urograffin 290 is a suitable contrast medium

EXAMINATION TWO

Allow 2 hours for the completion of all 60 questions
Answers are on page 79

2.1 Concerning radioactivity

A the specific activity of a radioactive source varies with temperature
B specific activity is measured as a percentage
C the half-life becomes shorter as radioactive decay proceeds
D β-decay involves the emission of a β particle from a K shell
E an α particle is equivalent to deuterium

2.2 Regarding the electromagnetic spectrum

A sound waves do not fall within the spectrum
B β emission falls in the short wavelength part of the spectrum
C visible light has a shorter wavelength than infrared
D the frequency and wavelength of ultraviolet light are directly proportional to each other
E the velocity of travel of radio waves in a vacuum is constant

2.3 Thermoluminescent dosimeters (TLD) for personal monitoring

A usually contain polytetrafluoroethylene (PTFE) in disc form
B the PTFE fluoresces when heated during measurement
C require annealing before being reused
D image fading occurs
E have a lower threshold than film badges in the diagnostic energy range

2.4 IRR 85 states the following dose limits

A 5 mSv to the whole body of a member of the public
B 150 mSv to the lens of the eye of a radiologist
C 50 mSv to the individual organs or tissues of a radiographer
D 10 mSv during any consecutive 3 month period to the abdomen of a woman of reproductive capacity
E 20 mSv per year averaged over 5 years, but no more than 50 mSv in a single year, to the whole body of a darkroom technician

2.5   The following are routinely indicated

A   a chest X-ray for pre-employment screening
B   an orbital radiograph for a metallic foreign body
C   a sacrococcygeal view for injury to the coccyx
D   a plain abdominal film for a lost intra-uterine contraceptive device
E   an intravenous urogram for microscopic haematuria

2.6   Regarding background radiation

A   the average annual total body dose in the UK is 2.5 mSv
B   medical radiation is the largest contributor to cancer induction in the UK
C   the greatest contribution is from inhaled air
D   in granite buildings it can exceed 50 mSv per year
E   in the UK, is highest in East Anglia

2.7   The intensity of an X-ray spectrum is increased by

A   increasing the kV across the tube
B   increasing the atomic number of the target
C   reducing the tube filtration
D   omitting the use of a focused grid
E   reducing the anode to cathode distance

2.8   Regarding filtration of X-rays

A   a molybdenum filter is an efficient filter of the characteristic radiation from a molybdenum anode
B   the half value layer increases with the linear attenuation coefficient
C   removing the tube filtration results in beam hardening
D   the orientation of a compound filter is unimportant
E   in the 70-100 kVp range the tube filtration should be at least 2.5 mm of aluminium

2.9   Regarding X-ray film processing

A   effective film speed can be increased by increasing development time
B   contrast is reduced by too great a replenishment rate of developer
C   fog is increased by the use of very acidic fixer
D   optical density increases with development time
E   film used in daylight systems is not sensitive to visible wavelengths

2.10 Regarding X-ray scatter

A grids can remove 100% of scatter
B reduced beam size reduces scatter
C reduced patient-film distance reduces scatter reaching the film
D scatter on an abdominal radiograph may be increased by the use of a patient compression band
E use of a scanning slit reduces scatter

2.11 Recording output of an image intensifier

A video recording imposes a vertical resolution limit due to the number of scan lines
B video recording does not affect image contrast
C TV/video gives images of lower resolution than those recorded on cine film
D cine film requires higher patient dose than conventional radiographs
E a half-silvered mirror is used to right the inverted image from the image intensifier

2.12 Regarding digital radiography

A digital image storage is not suitable for plain chest radiography
B image data can only be archived on optical disks
C contrast can be enhanced by digital processing
D mapping of digital data to image display is user-controlled
E displays of digital images can offer a maximum of 256 shades of grey

2.13 In computed tomography

A arrays of free air ionization chambers can be used for detection.
B a near monoenergetic beam is required for accurate image reconstruction.
C heavy filtration using copper or aluminium is used to reduce patient dose
D the image display usually contains 256, 512 or 1024 pixels
E the CT number (Hounsfield units) of each voxel in the slice has a range of 256

2.14 In ultrasound

A axial resolution refers to objects that lie at different distances from the transducer
B increasing the pulse repetition frequency increases the axial resolution
C the spatial pulse length must be less than twice the object separation in order to be resolved axially
D lateral and azimuthal resolution are equivalent
E the width of the beam must be less than the distance between the objects in order to be resolved laterally

2.15 Doppler shift from arterial blood

A is optimally detected with the transducer perpendicular to the vessel
B is optimally detected using a 3.5 MHz transducer
C duplex scanning refers to the combination of colour flow mapping and pulsed wave Doppler
D is at a maximum at the Nyquist frequency
E is maximally detected at twice the pulse repetition frequency

2.16 Regarding the static magnetic field in MRI

A superconducting magnets operate at liquid nitrogen temperatures (78 K)
B modern MRI equipment utilizes fields up to 0.2 Tesla
C metal instruments in the vicinity of the magnet are hazardous because of the heating effects of induced eddy currents
D MRI facilities are surrounded by a lead shield to prevent interference from and with external radiowaves
E the static field can cause heating of tissue

2.17 Regarding spin-echo pulse sequences in MRI

A a 90 degrees pulse is followed by a 180 degrees pulse after time TE
B the 180 degrees pulse neutralizes the effects of external field inhomogeneities
C T2 weighting is achieved by using a long TR and a long TE
D signal-to-noise ratio is increased by using a long TE
E TR refers to the time between the end of one pulse sequence and the start of the next

2.18 An ideal radiopharmaceutical should

A be a pure gamma emitter
B have a short biological half-life
C have a photon energy not exceeding 400 KeV
D be carrier free
E be colourless

2.19 In a gamma camera

A the scintillation crystals should have a high packing density
B crystals consist of sodium iodide doped with gallium
C the collimator lies adjacent to the photomultiplier tubes (PMT)
D the PMTs are triangular to improve spatial resolution
E the pulse height analyser generates X and Y coordinates

2.20 Regarding positron emission tomography (PET)

A PET involves the detection of gamma photons with energies in the range 100-400 keV
B PET utilizes positron-emitting radionuclides with long half-lives
C coincidence detection eliminates the need for lead collimators
D PET uses a single pair of detectors rotating around the patient
E positron emitters give a low patient dose

2.21 The following are branches of the internal carotid artery

A superficial temporal artery
B accessory meningeal artery
C pterygoid artery
D anterior choroidal artery
E posterior communicating artery

2.22 The following are correctly paired

A foramen ovale: middle meningeal artery
B jugular foramen: vagus nerve
C foramen spinosum: maxillary nerve
D greater palatine foramen: lingual artery
E foramen lacerum: glossopharyngeal nerve

2.23 The optic foramina

A have a maximum diameter of 6.5 mm in the majority of adults
B have a 'keyhole' appearance in up to 8% of the population
C lead to a canal up to 9 mm in length
D transmit the ophthalmic veins
E have a difference of up to 1 mm in diameter either side

2.24 The following are sites of normal intracranial calcification

A interclinoid ligament
B pacchonian bodies
C 4th ventricle
D dentate nucleus
E pituitary gland

2.25 The stomach

A receives all its blood supply from branches of the splenic artery
B has lymph drainage to the nodes around the head of pancreas
C is completely surrounded by peritoneum
D is related posteriorly to the left adrenal gland
E pyloric sphincter relaxation is inhibited by the right vagus

2.26 The pancreas

A lies on the splenic vein
B is completely retroperitoneal
C has two major ducts
D is related anteriorly to the lesser sac
E receives all its blood supply from the superior mesenteric artery

2.27 The ureters

A are retroperitoneal throughout their course
B are anterior to the gonadal arteries
C receive a blood supply from the renal artery
D lie on the psoas muscle
E are narrowed at the bifurcation of the common iliac arteries

2.28 The gallbladder

A may be absent
B contains within its neck the Spiral Valve of Heister
C is normally <9 cm in length on ultrasound measurement
D is supplied by a branch of the left hepatic artery
E has venous drainage directly into the hepatic vein

2.29 Concerning the thoracic aorta

A it gives rise to the right coronary artery from the posterior sinus
B the arch descends to the level of the 3rd thoracic vertebra
C the descending aorta has the left vagus nerve anterior and the left phrenic nerve posterior
D the ascending aorta is about 5 cm long
E it gives rise to the bronchial arteries in the majority

2.30 In a normal heart

A the mitral valve lies anteriorly to the aortic valve
B the aortic valve lies at the level of the 4th intercostal space
C the pulmonary valve is 3 cm in diameter
D the pulmonary valve lies at the apex of the conus arteriosus
E the tricuspid valve lies at the level of the 3rd intercostal space

2.31 At the level of the 4th thoracic vertebra

A the thoracic duct is posterior to the oesophagus
B the superior vena cava is formed
C the trachea has bifurcated
D the azygos vein is posterior to the oesophagus
E 1 cm diameter pre-tracheal lymph nodes are normally visible on transaxial CT scanning

2.32 The following structures are in direct contact with the diaphragm

A right kidney
B pancreas
C left adrenal gland
D spleen
E duodenal cap

2.33 **The navicular bone articulates with the following**

A 1st metatarsal
B lateral cunieform
C cuboid
D calcaneum
E talus

2.34 **In the pelvis**

A the sacroiliac joints are plane synovial joints
B the symphysis pubis is a plane synovial joint
C the maximum width of the symphysis pubis is 7 mm
D the inominate bone is composed of the ilium, ischium and pubis
E the sacrum has 10 foramina on its ventral surface

2.35 **Regarding the blood supply of the arm**

A the anterior circumflex humeral artery is a branch of the brachial artery
B the ulnar collateral artery supplies the elbow joint
C behind the pectoralis major the axillary artery is anterior to the radial nerve
D the cephalic vein is more medial than the basilic vein
E the axillary artery gives rise to the 1st and 2nd intercostal arteries

2.36 **Concerning the knee joint**

A it is supported by two intracapsular ligaments
B the fabella is situated on the postero-lateral margin of the knee
C the medial meniscus has a smaller diameter than the lateral in transverse section
D the anterior cruciate ligament tightens during knee flexion
E a coronary ligament attaches the medial meniscus to the tibia

2.37 In embryology

A normal midgut herniation into the umbilical cord occurs between 7 and 10 weeks

B external genitalia follow parallel lines of development until the 12th week

C the first ossification centre is in the clavicle

D the umbilical cord contains two veins and one artery

E the heart is derived from the mesoderm

2.38 In the brain

A the lentiform nucleus is composed of the putamen and the globus pallidus

B the great cerebral vein lies in the quadrigeminal cistern

C the third ventricle communicates with the fourth ventricle via the aqueduct of Sylvius

D the lateral ventricle communicates with the third ventricle via the foramen of Lushka

E the fourth ventricle communicates with the cisterna magna via the foramen of Munro

2.39 Concerning the fourth ventricle

A the roof is formed entirely by the cerebellar peduncles

B it lies behind the midbrain

C it contains choroid plexus

D medially it has the foramen of Magendie

E it is in direct communication with the cisterna magna

2.40 Regarding the nasolacrimal duct

A there is a constriction at the orbicularis oculi

B there is a constriction at the junction of the common canaliculus and the lacrimal sac

C it is approximately 4.5 cm in length

D it may normally be absent

E it drains into the inferior meatus

2.41 Regarding the gradient echo sequence in magnetic resonance scanning

A focal calcification cannot be demonstrated
B reducing the flip angle increases the T1 weighting
C field inhomogeneity is reduced in comparison to the spin echo sequence
D a proton dense image requires a flip angle of greater than 45 degrees
E at a constant flip angle, the T1 weighting is reduced if the TR is increased

2.42 Concerning ERCP

A a chest radiograph is desirable prior to the procedure
B an overcouch tube is preferable for screening
C the normal biliary tree requires 8-12 ml of contrast
D the normal pancreatic duct requires 6-8 ml of contrast
E most of the procedure is performed with the patient prone

2.43 Regarding lumbosacral myelography

A the injection is made with the patient upright
B the injection is made at the L3/4 intervertebral space
C the needle should not be moved once CSF is seen to drip from it
D the injection is observed under fluoroscopy
E the injection should be made over 30-60 seconds

2.44 Concerning lower limb venography

A superficial venous filling usually occurs because the needle has been inserted pointing away from the toes
B after unsuccessful venepuncture the needle should be removed and cannulation of a more proximal vein attempted
C a contrast media solution concentration of 350 mg iodine/ml is appropriate
D no more than 75 ml of contrast media solution should be injected
E a pump injector is preferred in order to reduce the radiation dose to the radiologist's hands

2.45 Regarding intravenous digital subtraction angiography (IV DSA)

A it usually requires an overnight stay in hospital
B it requires a central venous catheter
C images are obtained during the first pass of contrast medium
D the use of hyoscine-n-butyl bromide (buscopan) can improve image quality
E pixel-shifting degrades image quality

2.46 Concerning low osmolar iodinated contrast media

A iohexol (300 mg/ml) is iso-osmolar with plasma
B ioxaglate cannot be used in the spinal theca
C iotrolan is a non-ionic monomer
D they are never hypo-osmolar with respect to plasma
E they all do not ionize in solution

2.47 Regarding contrast media in computed tomography

A unopacified bowel contents have a similar Hounsfield number to other intrabdominal organs
B oral 2% gastrograffin is a useful agent for opacifying small bowel
C air can be a useful agent in pelvic scanning
D liver metastases maybe obscured during dynamic contrast enhancement
E scanning should be performed shortly after conventional myelography

2.48 The following are visible on a standard 30 degrees fronto-occipital skull radiograph

A saggital suture
B coronal suture above the lambdoid suture
C optic canal
D arcuate eminence of temporal bone
E mandibular condyle

2.49 Respiration is employed during exposure of the following radiographs

A lateral view of the thoracic spine
B anteroposterior view of the thoracic spine
C anteroposterior view of the thoracic inlet
D anteroposterior view of the diaphragm
E anteroposterior open mouth view of odontoid peg

2.50 Concerning radionuclide studies following myocardial infarction

A ^{99m} Tc DTPA is the most commonly used radiopharmaceutical
B there should be a delay of 8 hours after infarction prior to imaging
C uptake in ribs may give false positive results
D they are not reliable for the diagnosis of subendocardial infarcts
E the use of SPECT is an advantage

2.51 With a radionuclide bone scan

A no patient preparation is required
B ^{99m}Tc is the most commonly used isotope
C a typical effective dose equivalent is between 3 and 5 mSv
D the pedicles of normal lumbar vertebral bodies may be recognized
E the definition of long bones becomes less distinct with age

2.52 Regarding parotid sialography

A initially a sialogogue should be administered in order to identify the ductal orifice
B the catheter should be advanced at least 1.5 cm along the duct
C up to 0.75 ml of contrast is required in a healthy gland
D the injection is continued until the patient indicates it is causing pain
E after injection the syringe is taped on the forehead in the midline

2.53 Concerning a double contrast barium meal

A it requires no specific patient preparation
B the patient is rolled prone from the left lateral position in order to demonstrate gastro-oesophageal reflux
C in the supine LAO position the fundus and upper body of the stomach are seen in double contrast
D slightly depressing the head of the table from horizontal helps to demonstrate the duodenal cap
E an erect true lateral view is sometimes required

2.54 During a barium enema

A the caecum is best filled with barium by having the patient in a supine, table head up position

B Insufflation of air in the supine position will cause reflux through the ileocaecal valve

C excess barium in the rectum should be drained with the patient in the left lateral, table head up position

D balloon catheters are frequently useful in elderly patients

E the use of buscopan enhances the visualization of colonic haustra

2.55 Regarding CT myelography

A a greater dose of intrathecal contrast media is required than in conventional myelography

B it should only be performed if a conventional myelogram has given an equivocal result

C usually a small 'field of view' is used

D it should always be preceded by a conventional myelogram

E intrathecal contrast media is not always required to demonstrate nerve root compression

2.56 Concerning cranial magnetic resonance imaging

A unidentified bright objects (UBOs) are of high signal intensity on T_1 weighted images

B it is inferior in quality to CT in visualization of the contents of the posterior fossa

C it is as good as CT at demonstrating calcification

D intracerebral haemorrhage may not be detected in its early stages

E currently is of limited use in the acute management of severe head injuries

2.57 Concerning obstetric ultrasound

A thickening of the endometrium is a satisfactory confirmation of early pregnancy

B the pregnancy can only be said to be viable when fetal heart pulsations can be seen within the gestational sac

C the yolk sac lies outside the gestational sac

D fetal heart pulsations may first be seen at 5 to 6 weeks gestation with a transvaginal probe

E crown-rump length is useful for estimating gestational age from 10 to 15 weeks

2.58 Regarding transvaginal ultrasound

A two members of staff must be present
B it requires a full bladder
C it should be performed prior to the transabdominal ultrasound if a malignant mass is suspected
D the probe may be inserted by the patient
E it is advisable to wash the probe in Cidex following each examination

2.59 Concerning intravenous urography

A it requires thorough bowel preparation
B patients are fasted for 12 hours prior to the examination in order to improve the pyelographic density
C fluid restriction is contraindicated in patients with diabetes mellitus
D it should be avoided in patients with multiple myelomatosis
E image quality is improved when performed with the bladder full

2.60 Regarding retrograde pyelography

A it is contraindicated in the presence of urinary tract infection
B approximately 40 ml of contrast medium is required in a non-dilated system
C after the pelvicalyceal system is outlined the catheter is just withdrawn.
D if a ureteric obstruction is demonstrated, a delayed radiograph should be performed
E it is acceptable for patients to experience some loin pain

EXAMINATION THREE

Allow 2 hours for the completion of all 60 questions
Answers are on page 89

3.1 Concerning radioactivity

A a nuclide is an atom with a particular number of protons and neutrons
B isotopes of the same element may be separated by chemical methods
C radioactive decay occurs faster at higher temperatures
D radioactive decay of isotopes stored for long enough will eventually become exhausted
E the activity of a radioactive source is the mass that decays in unit time

3.2 Concerning the properties of X-rays

A the inverse square law is determined in part by the law of conservation of energy
B the inverse square law applies to X-rays emitted from a linear anode
C all electromagnetic radiation is ionizing
D X-rays have higher linear energy transfer than α particles
E X-rays may be produced by bombarding a tungsten anode with ultraviolet light

3.3 Regarding Compton scattering in the diagnostic range

A most scatter occurs in a forward direction
B there is more scatter on the tube side than the film side of the patient
C the X-ray photon has more energy than the recoil electron after scattering
D it occurs with unbound electrons
E it has an increased probability of occuring as X-ray photon energy increases

3.4 Regarding statutory responsibilities

A the Ionising Radiation Regulations 1985 are governed by the principle of 'as low as reasonably achievable' (ALARA)

B the Ionising Radiation Regulations 1988 are often referred to as the 'POPUMET' regulations

C radioisotopes can only be administered by someone who holds the 'core of knowledge' or IRR 88 certificate

D Administration of Radioactive Substances Advisory Committee (ARSAC) licence is granted to the health authority or trust

E Crown immunity exempts all NHS hospitals in the UK from the regulations governing the storage of radioactive materials

3.5 Concerning radiation protection

A radiation protection advisors normally reside in an X-ray department.

B the radiation protection committee should have a representative of the hospital administration on it

C a GP who requests a chest X-ray is clinically directing the examination

D a radiographer who performs a chest X-ray is physically directing the examination

E during pacemaker wire insertion, the clinician who operates the footswitch is only clinically directing the examination

3.6 Non-stochastic effects include

A leukaemia

B infertility

C bone marrow ablation

D ankylosing spondylitis

E skin erythema

3.7 Regarding the spatial distribution of X-rays

A the anode heel effect is due to some radiation being absorbed within the target

B the anode heel effect occurs more on the cathode side of the tube

C the larger the anode angle the larger the anode heel effect

D extra focal radiation refers to X-rays produced at the periphery of the target

E extra focal radiation can be as much as 50% of the total output of the tube

3.8   X-ray tube rating increases with

A   increasing focal spot size
B   stationary compared with rotating anodes
C   full wave compared with half wave rectification
D   slow dissipation of heat from the anode
E   increasing anode angle for a fixed focal spot size

3.9   Intensifying screens are used to

A   reduce patient dose
B   increase image sharpness
C   improve image contrast
D   reduce electricity costs
E   remove scattered radiation

3.10   Optical density of X-ray film

A   is the ratio of the incident and reflected light intensities
B   must be considered in order to assess the contrast of a film
C   is zero when the film is unexposed
D   usefully lies between 0.25 and 1.0 for X-ray film
E   of two films is the sum of their individual optical densities

3.11   Concerning latitude, gamma and speed of X-ray film

A   a wide range of crystal sizes in the emulsion gives a low gamma
B   a film with a low gamma has a wide exposure latitude
C   a faster film requires higher exposure factors to produce the same
    density
D   a slow film gives a less 'grainy' image
E   a fast emulsion has a small gamma

3.12   In computed tomography

A   spatial resolution is superior to conventional radiography
B   contrast resolution is inferior to conventional radiography over the
    whole contrast range
C   noise level is directly proportional to slice thickness
D   noise level increases as pixel size decreases
E   contrast resolution is improved in thicker slices

3.13 Regarding conventional tomography

A zonography involves very small angles between the slice and the axis of the detector

B zonography gives thick slices

C large angle tomography gives thin slices and high contrast resolution

D movement of both X-ray tube and film is essential

E wide angle tomography requires shorter exposure times

3.14 Regarding ultrasound

A the time gain compensator (TGC) enhances near echoes

B the near gain and far gain work as part of the TGC

C the overall gain works as part of the TGC

D all reflected echoes are displayed on the screen

E enhancement from a region of interest requires the TGC

3.15 Ultrasound can cause injury

A by heating

B by streaming

C by cavitation

D by ionization

E when used above a threshold SPTA intensity of $100 \, \text{mW/cm}^2$

3.16 Magnetic resonance imaging

A is concerned with the magnetic moments of spinning nuclear particles

B can only be carried out on nuclei with no orbiting electrons

C can only be carried out on hydrogen nuclei

D can only be carried out on nuclei with an odd number of protons or neutrons

E detects magnetic moments associated with spinning electron clouds

3.17 Regarding transverse magnetization in MRI

A transverse magnetization decreases to zero in time T2

B transverse magnetization is caused by magnetic moments precessing in phase with each other

C transverse magnetization decreases as energy is transferred to the surrounding lattice

D inhomogeneities in the external field tend to decrease transverse magnetization

E the transverse relaxation time (T2) is always less than T1 in biological tissue

3.18 Regarding tissue characteristics in MRI

A water has a long T2 because of a high degree of inhomogeneity in the magnetic field

B fat has a short T1 and a short T2

C the presence of impurities dissolved in water tends to increase T2

D paramagnetic contrast media tend to increase T1 and T2 in their surroundings

E proton densities of soft tissues show greater variation than the corresponding T1 relaxation times

3.19 Technetium-99m

A is a pure gamma emitter

B is not easily bound to biologically relevant molecules

C emits monoenergetic 511 keV gamma rays

D has a biological half-life of 6 hours

E decays to Mo-99

3.20 Regarding a gamma camera

A the crystal is hermetically sealed to prevent escape of radioactive material

B the minimum count rate that can be detected is limited by the dead time of the system

C the sensitivity of the system decreases above count rates of 2×10^4 counts per minute

D a useful image cannot be formed without the use of a collimator

E output signals from the gamma camera can be fed directly to a digital computer

3.21 The following are correctly paired

A foramen magnum: temporal bone
B superior orbital fissure: sphenoid bone
C carotid canal: occipital bone
D foramen spinosum: temporal bone
E foramen rotundum: petrous bone

3.22 Calcification can occur normally in the following sites

A pineal gland
B pituitary gland
C red nucleus
D tentorium
E interclinoid ligament

3.23 The parotid gland contains the following

A external carotid artery
B internal carotid artery
C inferior ophthalmic artery
D facial nerve
E inferior alveolar nerve

3.24 Concerning the spine

A the distance between the tips of the transverse processes of a vertebral body is greatest at L4
B the spinous process of C6 is the most easily palpable in the cervical spine
C the inferior border of the scapula is opposite T6
D the vertebral artery enters the vertebral foramen at C6
E variations in usual the number of thoracic, lumbar and sacral vertebrae occur in 5% of the population

3.25 Concerning the right kidney

A the hilum lies at the level of L4
B the most anterior hilar vessel is the renal artery
C a renal artery may normally pass posterior to the pelvis of the ureter
D it is covered anteriorly by the 2nd part of the duodenum
E a length of 10 cm is normal

3.26 The coeliac axis

A can give rise to the superior mesenteric artery
B has two main branches
C supplies all the structures derived from the foregut
D is about 5 cm long
E supplies the lower third of the oesophagus

3.27 Regarding the liver

A it normally weighs about 1 kg in an adult
B is attached to the anterior abdominal wall and diaphragm by three peritoneal folds
C it arises as a ventral outgrowth of the foregut into the ventral mesentery
D the left lobe is in contact with the oesophagus
E it has a fibrous capsule

3.28 The following are branches of the internal iliac artery

A umbilical artery
B internal pudendal artery
C middle rectal artery
D right testicular artery
E appendicular artery

3.29 The thoracic duct

A is about 25 cm long
B passes anterior to the oesophagus at the level of T5
C passes through the diaphragm at T10
D passes behind the carotid sheath at the level of C7
E usually drains into the left subclavian vein

3.30 The following empty directly into the right atrium

A the great cardiac vein
B the coronary sinus
C the anterior cardiac veins
D the oblique vein of the left atrium
E venae cordis minimae

3.31 Regarding the lobes of the lungs

  A the left lung is composed of three lobes in 10% of adults
  B an azygos 'lobe' is present in less than 1% of adults
  C the right lung contains 10 bronchopulmonary segments
  D the posterior basal segment of the right lower lobe lies adjacent to the right heart border
  E the lingular bronchi arise directly from the left main bronchus

3.32 Concerning the thoracic cage

  A the 1st rib has only one articular facet on its head
  B the 12th rib has no subcostal grove
  C the heads of the 2nd to 12th ribs have two facets for articulation
  D all vertebrae have three centres of secondary ossification
  E on a PA chest radiograph the transverse processes of T1 point caudally

3.33 The ossification centres in the elbow appear in the following order

  A capitellum: 1st
  B trochlear: 3rd
  C olecranon: 5th
  D medial epicondyle: 4th
  E lateral epicondyle: 6th

3.34 In the ankle

  A Bohler's angle is between 28 and 40 degrees
  B the maximum male heel pad thickness is <21.5 mm
  C the os vesalianum lies adjacent to the navicular
  D the deltoid ligament attaches to the talus
  E the lateral ligament attaches to the calcaneus

3.35 Concerning the arteries of the leg

  A the profunda femoral artery is more medial than the superficial femoral artery
  B the superficial epigastric artery arises from the femoral artery below the inguinal ligament
  C the peroneal artery is a branch of the anterior tibial artery
  D the medial circumflex femoral artery is a branch of the profunda femoral artery
  E the dorsalis pedis is the terminal branch of the anterior tibial artery

3.36 The shoulder joint

A is supported by three glenohumeral ligaments
B is a ball and socket synovial joint
C is closely related to the axillary nerve
D only has one third of the humeral head in the glenoid labrum
E relies more on muscles than ligaments for support

3.37 Concerning the subarachnoid cisterns

A the prepontine cistern lies between the pons and the clivus
B the prepontine cistern contains the basilar artery
C the quadrigemnal cistern contains the great vein of Galen
D the suprasellar cistern contains the optic nerves
E the ambient cistern contains the anterior but not the posterior choroidal arteries

3.38 The uterus

A is normally up to 8 cm long
B is supported by the round ligament
C is fully retroperitoneal
D has a blood supply from the ovarian artery
E is attached to two fallopian tubes 6 cm long

3.39 The sinuses open at the following sites

A frontal sinus: middle meatus
B sphenoid sinus: sphenoid-ethmoid recess
C maxillary antrum: inferior meatus
D nasolacrimal duct: middle meatus
E eustachian tube: the lateral nasopharyngeal wall

3.40 Concerning the pharnyx

A all the muscles are supplied by the vagus nerve
B it receives sensory supply from the trigeminal nerve
C it is supplied by the external carotid artery
D it has three sets of constrictor muscles
E it extends to the level of C6

3.41 Concerning peroperative cholangiography

A images of surgical instruments should not appear on the radiographs
B urograffin 150 is a suitable contrast agent
C the injection is made with the patient supine
D a single hand injection should be performed
E the radiographs should be immediately reported by a radiologist

3.42 Regarding lumbosacral myelography

A kV of 90 is appropriate for the AP and oblique views
B a grid is required for all radiographs
C the initial radiographs are taken with the patient prone
D with an overcouch tube it is the left nerve roots that are demonstrated in the LPO position
E a lateral radiograph is always required

3.43 Concerning lower limb venography

A non-ionic contrast should always be used
B a film showing the initial filling is valuable
C the foot should always be included in the study
D a Valsalva manoeuvre is performed in order to maintain contrast media in the leg
E if a thrombus is demonstrated the limb should not be exercized

3.44 Hyoscine-n-butyl bromide should be used with caution in patients with

A open angle glaucoma
B thyrotoxicosis
C renal colic
D prostatic enlargement
E cardiac failure

3.45 Concerning intravenous digital subtraction angiography (IV DSA)

A image acquisition commences as contrast medium administration is occurring
B low osmolar contrast media should always be used
C it is contra-indicated when there is a history of pulmonary embolism
D it is valuable in the diagnosis of renal artery stenosis
E can be used in children

3.46 Regarding iodinated ionic and non-ionic contrast media

A during an intravenous urogram (IVU), the pyelogram is denser with an ionic agent

B during an IVU distension of the collecting system is improved with an ionic agent

C non-ionic agents have a stronger anticoagulant action

D the stated mortality from an adverse reaction to an ionic agent is 1:40 000

E they are safe for use in pregnancy

3.47 Gadolinium DTPA

A shortens T_1 and T_2 relaxation times

B is a stable chelate

C is directly visualized during imaging

D is administered in a dose of 0.5 mmol/kg

E is mainly excreted in bile

3.48 The radiographic centring points and beam angulation for the following cranial radiographs are correct

A a submento-vertical view of the skull: midway between the angles of the mandible

B 20 degrees occipitofrontal view of the skull: the nasion through the occipital bone

C right lateral oblique view of the mandible: 5 cm below the angle of the mandible nearest to the film

D 30 degrees occipito-mental view of the face: lower orbital margin though the skull vertex

E 30 degrees fronto-occipital view of the skull: foramen magnum through the frontal bone

3.49 During a postero-anterior oblique view of the cervical spine

A the patient may be sitting or standing

B gonad protection should be employed

C the median saggital plane of the skull should be parallel to the film

D 15 degrees of cranial angulation is used

E the intervertebral foramina nearest the film are demonstrated

3.50 Regarding thallium-201 myocardial imaging

A ^{201}Tl thallous chloride is a useful radiopharmaceutical
B ^{201}Tl is distributed according to regional blood flow
C no patient preparation is required
D myocardial stress is an integral part of the study
E it can be used to monitor the result of a coronary angioplasty

3.51 The uptake of ^{99m}Tc pertechnetate following intravenous injection is normal in

A gastric parietal cells
B the sublingual salivary glands
C the scrotum
D the sweat glands
E the lacrimal glands and ducts

3.52 Concerning submandibular sialography

A it is more often successful than parotid sialography
B the orifice of the duct should be identified by external massage
C an indication of pain by the patient is an unreliable sign that the gland has been properly opacified
D digital or photographic subtraction optimizes the technique
E it may result in death

3.53 A small bowel enema

A may be used to determine the site of intestinal obstruction
B uses a modified Bilbao-Dotter tube
C takes less time to complete than a barium follow-through examination
D requires colonic preparation
E requires an overnight fast prior to the examination

3.54 Regarding positioning during a barium enema

A the prone oblique projection is primarily used to prevent overlapping of the sigmoid colon and rectum
B a true lateral view is obligatory
C the hepatic flexure is best seen in a LAO position
D the splenic flexure usually requires a greater degree of obliquity than the hepatic flexure to be optimally visualized
E the transverse colon is seen in double contrast with the patient prone

3.55 Concerning CT scanning in children

A written parental consent is required for non-urgent scans
B it is desirable for a parent or nurse to accompany the child in the scan room
C it is mainly performed for the investigation of epilepsy
D abdominal scans are generally more difficult to interpret than those of adults
E the lungs should be examined under general anaesthesia

3.56 Measurements made on an ultrasound monitor screen

A should not be made with sector scanning transducers
B should be made perpendicular to the direction of the beam if possible
C should generally be made between the leading edge of a near surface and the trailing edge of a distant surface
D those of the common bile duct should be made from its inner border to inner border
E those of the common hepatic duct (CHD) are made where the hepatic artery crosses between the portal vein and the CHD itself

3.57 Concerning obstetric ultrasound and gestational age estimation

A bi-parietal diameter (BPD) may be used when the lie is breech
B when measuring femoral length, the furthest of two visible femurs should be measured
C soft tissue should be visible at each end of a femur being measured
D when measuring BPD, a midline stripe should be seen continuously from front to back of the head
E BPD and femoral length measurement are equally accurate

3.58 Regarding intravenous urography

A control radiographs are exposed at a low kilovoltage
B a control film maybe omitted if a KUB radiograph has been performed on the same day
C an anxious patient is more likely to have an adverse reaction to contrast media
D gonad protection should be used in males
E a lateral radiograph maybe required to demonstrate renal position

3.59 Micturating cystography

A may be used to demonstrate vesicovaginal fistulae
B is contraindicated in the presence of urinary tract infection
C may be performed if the patient is an asthmatic
D may be performed with or without bladder catheterization
E looking for vesico-ureteric reflux requires bladder catheterization

3.60 Regarding ascending urethrography

A the Whitaker apparatus is useful
B a catheter should be inserted into the posterior urethra and withdrawn while contrast medium is injected
C urograffin 150 is a suitable contrast medium
D it is useful for demonstrating the posterior urethra
E oblique radiographs should be taken with the legs extended

EXAMINATION FOUR

Allow 2 hours for the completion of all 60 questions
Answers are on page 97

4.1 The photoelectric effect

A is most important at the high end of the diagnostic range of energies
B results in the emission of continuous radiation
C is a pure absorption process in biological tissues
D varies with the square of the atomic number of the target
E concerns free electrons

4.2 Concerning attenuation of X-rays

A scattered X-rays will be completely eliminated if enough barium plaster is used on the walls
B linear attenuation coefficient increases with increasing density
C mass attenuation coefficient is independent of density
D absorption is the sum of attenuation and scatter
E the half value layer for water is about 60 mm in the diagnostic range of energies

4.3 Regarding radiation damage

A non-stochastic (deterministic) effects occur above a certain threshold
B the risk of a stochastic effect for a large group depends on the magnitude of the dose received
C stochastic effects are a more important consideration than non-stochastic (deterministic) effects in diagnostic radiology
D stochastic effects occur due to DNA and chromosomal damage
E all stochastic effects cause harm

4.4 Concerning personal doses

A workers who receive less than 30% of a dose limit cannot be classified
B a nurse who works permanently in an X-ray department is usually classified
C the radiation dose records of a classified worker must be kept for 2 years
D personal monitoring badges must be worn by all unclassified radiologists performing fluoroscopy
E the ALARA principle applies to occupational dose as well as patient dose

4.5 During fluoroscopy the equipment malfunctions

A effective dose is best estimated using a dose area product meter
B a dose area product meter is attached beneath the patient when using overcouch screening
C effective dose can be measured directly
D male gonad dose can be estimated by attaching a thermoluminescent dosemeter (TLD) to the scrotum
E the Health and Safety Executive must be informed if the actual exposure is twice the intended

4.6 Concerning radiographic examination

A the patient has the prime responsibility for declaring her pregnancy just prior to radiography
B consulting patients notes is a reliable method of determining previous X-ray examination
C computed tomography makes the largest man-made contribution to collective dose in the UK
D dental films are performed more frequently than chest X-rays in the UK
E using the 28 day rule may result in a pregnant woman being radiographed

4.7 The quality of an X-ray beam is affected by

A kVp
B filtration
C voltage waveform
D shape of the anode
E tube current

4.8 Unsharpness in radiology is reduced by

A increasing the speed of anode rotation
B increasing the thickness of the screen phosphor
C using pigment in the screen phosphor
D using double emulsion film
E increasing the anode angle

4.9 Regarding intensifying screen-film combinations

A rare earth screens are reserved for special applications in most modern X-ray departments
B screens consist of a single large crystal bound on to a metallic or paper substrate
C efficiency is measured by the intensifying factor
D screens are usually made of sodium iodide
E screens have a high atomic number

4.10 Concerning the characteristic curve of screen-film combination

A increasing exposure can result in a decrease in film density
B the gamma is measured in the shoulder region of the curve
C exposure is plotted on a linear scale
D it changes shape when an intensifying screen is used
E it indicates a finite density when an exposure has not been made

4.11 In computed tomography

A in Hounsfield units, air has a CT number of zero
B the window level refers to the lowest CT number displayed
C contrast is enhanced by using a narrow window width
D beam hardening artefacts can show as an increase in density in the centre of a uniform object
E doubling spatial resolution results in a four-fold increase in patient dose

4.12 Regarding X-ray grids

A grids remove scattered rays without reducing primary beam intensity
B grids increase patient dose
C grids consist of lead strips separated by air
D grid ratio is the ratio of the height of the lead strips to their width
E contrast improvement factor (K) is the ratio of contrast with the grid to that without the grid

4.13 Diagnostic ultrasound

A has a frequency of greater than 20 kHz
B the particles oscillate in a direction perpendicular to the direction of the wave
C has a velocity of approximately 1450 m/sec in human soft tissue
D intensity is measured in decibels
E intensity is usually measured at spatial peak, temporal average when considering potential tissue damage

4.14 Regarding ultrasound

A the machine spends more time receiving than transmitting sound waves
B the pulse repetition frequency is equal to the frequency of the sound wave
C in pulsed ultrasound only sound of a single frequency is transmitted
D continuous wave ultrasound requires separate transmitting and receiving transducers
E bandwidth and pulse duration are not related

4.15 Regarding the MR signal

A tranverse magnetization is measured in preference to longitudinal magnetization
B the signal maybe detected by the same coils used to produce the RF pulse
C the frequency of the signal can give spatial information about its source
D the magnitude of the signal increases as the longitudinal magnetization returns to its original value
E the signal has a frequency in the range 10-200 kHz

4.16 Regarding contrast in MRI

A in a T2 spin-echo sequence, contrast is increased by increasing TE
B paramagnetic contrast media increase tissue contrast at the cost of increased imaging times
C T1 weighting is the preferred technique after contrast medium injection
D paramagnetic contrast media shorten relaxation times of the surrounding nuclei
E proton density images show little contrast between bone and soft tissue

4.17 Potential hazards associated with MRI include

A generation of a potential difference in flowing blood
B interference with cardiac pacemakers
C haemorrhage due to forces imposed on ferromagnetic plates or other implants
D significant cumulative radiation doses to staff
E burning due to careless handling of liquid helium and nitrogen

4.18 Regarding spatial resolution of a gamma camera

A intrinsic resolution is determined primarily by the size of the PMTs
B system resolution can be improved by use of a pinhole collimator
C spatial resolution increases with the thickness of the crystal
D system resolution is of the order of 1-2 mm
E spatial resolution is measured using a flood phantom

4.19 Regarding dynamic imaging with radioisotopes

A regions of interest must be selected prior to renogram scanning
B deconvolution involves mathematical treatment of image data to compensate for background counts
C renographic studies place the most stringent demands on a gamma camera
D electrocardiographic gating allows a longer scan time for cardiac studies
E renograms involve maximum frame rates of one per minute

4.20 Regarding SPECT

A gives superior resolution to conventional CT
B camera non-uniformities produce ring artefacts
C improved resolution is given by rotating the gamma camera in an eliptical orbit
D signal to noise ratio is higher than for planar imaging
E only provides transaxial sections

4.21 In a normal skull

    A calcification in the Habenular commisure lies anterior to the pineal
    B the ethmoid bone forms part of the nasal septum
    C the ethmoid bone articulates with the palatine bone
    D the vertebral arteries are the same size in the majority
    E the frontal sinuses open into the superior meatus

4.22 In a normal spine

    A the cervical nerves exit from foramina above the corresponding vertebral bodies
    B the atlas has no foramina transversaria
    C the spinous process of C2-6 are bifid
    D spina bifida occulta is present in up to 10% of the population
    E in the majority, the artery of Adamkiewicz arises from the right lumbar artery

4.23 Regarding the cranial nerves

    A the 4th supplies the medial rectus
    B the 12th supplies all the muscles of the tongue except mylohyoid
    C the facial nerve carries only motor fibres
    D the 6th cranial nerve is the only one to arise from the posterior brain stem
    E the 5th cranial nerve emerges from the midbrain

4.24 Concerning the cavernous sinus

    A the lateral wall contains five nerves
    B it is related to the temporal lobe of the brain
    C it drains to the pterygoid plexus
    D it is traversed by the anterior cerebral artery
    E its roof is continuous with the diaphragma sella

4.25 Regarding the suprarenal glands

    A the right gland lies adjacent to the diaphragm
    B they are each supplied by two arteries
    C they each have a single drainage vein
    D they are 5 cm in length
    E seen from the front, the right gland is crescentic in shape

4.26 Concerning the peritoneal spaces

A the lesser sac communicates via the foramen of Winslow with the right subhepatic space

B the left subhepatic space is bounded on the right by the falciform ligament

C the lesser sac contains the common bile duct

D the right lateral paracolic gutter communicates with the pelvic cavity

E right infracolic space communicates directly with the pelvic cavity

4.27 Regarding the liver

A the quadrate lobe is supplied by the right hepatic artery

B the caudate lobe is supplied by the left hepatic artery

C the ligamentum teres lies in the edge of the falciform ligament

D the hepatic artery arises from the left gastric artery in about 10% of people

E the hepatic veins converge on the bare areas of the liver

4.28 Concerning the colon

A the ileocaecal valve is incompetent in 65% of patients

B the transverse colon is retroperitoneal

C it is usually less than 1 m long in an adult

D it may normally have appendices epiploicae present

E the sigmoid arteries are derived from the inferior mesenteric artery

4.29 The right pulmonary artery

A measures up to 25 mm in diameter in an adult male

B is posterior to the superior vena cava

C increases in diameter on inspiration

D is contained within the serous pericardium

E is in close relation to the thoracic duct

4.30 The following are tributaries of the azygos vein

A right ascending lumbar vein

B right bronchial veins

C internal thoracic vein

D 4th right posterior intercostal vein

E hemiazygos vein

4.31 Concerning the blood supply of the normal heart

A the right coronary artery supplies the atrioventricular node
B the anterior intraventricular artery is a branch of the right coronary artery
C the great cardiac vein drains the territory supplied by the right coronary artery
D the circumflex artery is a branch of the left coronary artery
E the pericardium derives its blood supply from the internal thoracic artery

4.32 The following may normally indent the oesophagus

A cricopharyngeus muscle
B left atrium
C left main bronchus
D left ventricle
E anterior ascending aorta

4.33 The following ligaments connect the atlas to the axis

A alar ligament
B cruciform ligament
C membrane tectoria
D apical ligament
E anterior longitudinal ligament

4.34 Regarding the femoral triangle

A it is bordered laterally by sartorius
B the femoral nerve is lateral to the femoral artery
C contains deep lymph nodes within the femoral canal
D contains the femoral artery which enters the triangle under the midpoint of a line between the anterior superior iliac spine and the symphysis pubis
E has the great saphenous opening anteriorly

4.35 The exit foramina of the following cranial nerves are correct

A 2nd: optic foramen
B maxillary nerve: foramen rotundum
C 6th: optic foramen
D 10th: jugular foramen
E 11th: hypoglossal canal

4.36 Concerning the testes

A they receive a nerve supply from the 10th thoracic segment
B they are separated by a median scrotal septum
C the left testicular vein drains into the internal iliac vein
D they are supplied by a branch of the internal iliac artery
E they share lymphatic drainage with the scrotal skin

4.37 The pituitary fossa

A has a maximum AP diameter of 12 mm on a lateral skull radiograph
B has a dorsum sellae which lies anteriorly
C lies in close relation to the sphenoid sinus
D lies in relation to the cavernous sinus
E cannot be seen on a Townes projection

4.38 The temperomandibular joint

A is supported by two ligaments
B has the lateral pterygoid ligament attached to the inferior aspect of the joint
C is a synovial joint
D receives blood from the superficial temporal artery
E the condyle but not the articular disc move when the mouth is opened

4.39 Concerning the 8 segments of the liver

A 1st segment is the caudate lobe
B 2nd, 3rd and 4th segments form the right lobe of liver
C each bile duct and segmental artery lie medial to the segmental vein
D all lobes drain to the hepatic veins
E 4th segment is bordered by the falciform ligament

4.40 **The following are parts of the femur**

A quadrate tubercle
B linea aspera
C spiral line
D greater trochanter
E inferior gluteal line

4.41 **Regarding peroperative cholangiography**

A the common bile duct diameter should not exceed 12 mm
B free flow of contrast into the duodenum should be seen on all radio-graphs
C the terminal narrow segment of the duct should always be demon-strated
D a single filling defect in the biliary system is normal
E spasm of the sphincter of Oddi is not relieved by glucagon

4.42 **Regarding thoracic (dorsal) myelography**

A contrast medium requirements are the same as for lumbar myelography
B the bolus of contrast is run up from the lumbar spine with the patient supine
C movement of the contrast medium should be observed using fluoros-copy
D about 30 degrees of head down tilt are required in order to shift the contrast to the mid thoracic spine
E oblique views are not usually required

4.43 **Concerning intraosseous pelvic venography**

A it is only indicated when direct venepuncture is not possible
B it should be performed under general anaesthesia in infants
C a Potts-Cournand needle is used
D contrast media is injected into the iliac wing
E the internal iliac veins are demonstrated in the supine position

4.44 **Concerning hyoscine-n-butyl bromide**

A it may be mixed with aqueous contrast media
B the adult dose is 10 mg IM/IV
C it has an immediate onset of action
D its use requires special advice to outpatients
E it antagonizes insulin

4.45 **Regarding intrarterial digital subtraction angiography (IA DSA)**

A   spatial resolution is superior to conventional angiography
B   contrast resolution is superior to conventional angiography
C   catheterization technique and contrast media requirements are the same as for conventional angiography
D   buscopan can be administered directly through the arterial catheter
E   it is useful for imaging the portal venous system

4.46 **Low osmolar water soluble contrast agents may be used in the paediatric gastrointestinal tract if**

A   bronchial aspiration is possible
B   there is a distal small bowel or colonic obstruction
C   treatment of meconium ileus or milk inspissation is needed
D   demonstration of gastroesophageal reflux is required
E   the child has coeliac disease

4.47 **Gadolinium DTPA**

A   is a superparamagnetic substance
B   is safer than contrast enhanced CT when used in MR scanning
C   may induce epileptic seizures
D   is not recommended for patients below 18 years of age
E   is safe in pregnancy

4.48 **The following radiographic centring points are correct**

A   dorsipalmar oblique view of the hand: head of the fifth metacarpal
B   lateral view of the wrist: radial styloid process
C   anteroposterior view of right elbow: midway between the epicondyles of the humerus
D   anteroposterior view of the shoulder: coracoid process
E   inferosuperior view of the clavicle: midshaft of the clavicle

4.49 **Regarding a high kVp chest radiograph**

A   the air gap technique may be employed
B   a decreased FFD may be required
C   the skin dose is lower than a 65 kVp chest radiograph
D   it is useful for optimally demonstrating pulmonary calcification
E   it frequently shows the anterior junction line

4.50 Concerning radionuclide studies of the lung

A ^{99m}Tc DTPA can be used for a ventilation scan
B the injection should be made during arrested respiration
C less than 0.5% of the capillary bed is embolized during a perfusion scan
D ^{99m}Tc macroaggregated albumin (MAA) is contraindicated in patients with right to left cardiac shunts
E a perfusion scan alone can exclude pulmonary embolism

4.51 High uptake on a ^{99m}Tc MDP bone scan may be seen in

A calcification in costal cartilages
B the chest wall of patients with cardiac pacemakers
C the epiphyses of children
D the right shoulder of a right handed person
E the foot of a patient with prostatism

4.52 Barium swallow is indicated for

A odynophagia
B initial assessment of the reanastomosis following oesophago-gastrectomy
C achalasia
D bolus displacement of a foreign body
E suspected hiatus hernia

4.53 Regarding a small bowel enema

A there are no absolute contraindications to the procedure
B it is useful for the investigation of recurrent bleeding from the gastrointestinal tract
C it is likely to convert a small bowel obstruction from partial to complete by barium impaction
D it is the investigation of choice in coeliac disease
E iodinated water soluble contrast is preferred in the investigation of jejunal diverticulosis

4.54 Regarding a colostomy barium enema

A standard oral preparation is sufficient
B a normal rectal tube is appropriate
C a smooth muscle relaxant is strongly advisable
D air is insufflated with the patient on his left side
E flexural views are taken with the patient erect

4.55 Magnetic resonance imaging

A may be used to demonstrate placenta praevia
B should be avoided in the investigation of intraocular foreign bodies
C is contraindicated in the presence of intracranial aneurysm clips
D may be unsuitable for the obese
E the cardiac arrest team may not enter the scan room even in an emergency

4.56 Concerning hepatobiliary ultrasound

A no patient preparation is necessary
B the left lobe of the liver is preferably examined intercostally
C it can be normal for the liver and right kidney to be of equal echogenicity
D bile ducts run parallel to portal vein branches
E the normal CBD dilates after a fatty meal

4.57 In ultrasound foetal anatomy

A the choroid plexus is echo poor
B the thalamus is echo poor
C the fourth ventricle is routinely seen beneath the cerebellum
D the anterior horn of the lateral ventricle and the insula are easily confused
E the thalamus, cisterna magna and cerebellum may be seen on the same view

4.58   Regarding intravenous urography

A   approximately 300 mg of iodine per kilogram of body weight is appropriate for adults with unimpaired renal function
B   patients with renal impairment should have the dose of iodine reduced
C   the nephrogram is due largely to filtered contrast in the proximal convoluted tubules
D   nephrographic density is reduced if the patient is overhydrated
E   differing nephrographic density may be due to overlying bowel shadow

4.59   Regarding micturating cystography in adults

A   a 16F Foley catheter is appropriate
B   urograffin 150 is a suitable contrast medium
C   usually at least 200 ml of contrast media are required to fill the bladder
D   micturition should be performed in the erect position
E   oblique radiographs are required to optimally demonstrate vesico-ureteric reflux

4.60   Hysterosalpingography

A   may be used to confirm tubal occlusion after laparoscopic sterilization
B   can be performed in the presence of endometrial carcinoma
C   optimally should be performed during the seventh to tenth days of a regular menstrual cycle
D   may require pethidine to relieve painful tubal spasm
E   requires the presence of a gynaecologist

EXAMINATION FIVE

Allow 2 hours for the completion of all 60 questions
Answers are on page 105

5.1 Concerning atomic structure

A Z of $^{15}_{32}$P is equal to 15
B A of $^{15}_{32}$P is equal to 47
C Z is equal to the number of neutrons in the nucleus
D A is equal to the number of neutrons and protons in the nucleus
E Z determines an element's place in the periodic table

5.2 Regarding absorption edges

A an absorption edge occurs when the X-ray photon has slightly less energy than the electrons in the electron shell
B mass absorption coefficient decreases continuously as X-ray photon energy increases
C K absorption edges are not important in mammography
D barium has a K edge outside of the main energies of the beam
E for the same range of X-ray energy a material of low atomic number can never have a higher mass absorption coefficient than one of high atomic number

5.3 Regarding radioactivity

A nuclides may emit more than one type of radiation
B γ-rays are emitted with a continuous range of energies
C γ-emitters are more harmful if ingested than α-emitters as the radiations are more penetrating
D half-life is directly proportional to decay constant
E a positron and an electron can annihilate to form electromagnetic radiation

5.4 Concerning radiation protection

A equivalent doses allow a range of non-uniform organ doses to be combined as a single number
B the radiation weighting factor (ICRP 60) is the same for α particles and γ-rays
C X-rays have a radiation weighting factor of unity
D absorbed dose and equivalent dose are numerically equivalent for diagnostic range X-rays
E alpha particles have a higher linear energy transfer than high energy neutrons (>20 MeV)

5.5 Concerning annual whole body doses

A most health workers receive less than 1 mSv per year
B for radiographers are usually higher than for radiologists
C for radiologists are usually higher than for cardiologists who perform screening
D limits are defined in IRR 88 for patients whilst undergoing radiographic examination
E patients in an X-ray departmental waiting area are regarded as members of the public

5.6 Regarding staff protection

A the heaviest tolerable lead apron should be worn
B aprons have a lead equivalent of 1.25 to 1.5 mm
C lead aprons afford adequate protection from the primary beam
D lead gloves afford adequate protection from the primary beam
E a standard lead apron will transmit less than 10% of the incident energy at 100 kV

5.7 Concerning mammography

A mammography should be performed on a woman with long-standing nipple inversion
B mammography should be performed routinely prior to hormone replacement therapy
C there is twice the risk of fatal breast cancer induction, in women between 30 and 49 than those between 50 and 65, for a single view mammogram
D the NHS screening programme invites women between 50 and 64 every 5 years for a mammogram
E sensitivity is reduced in the young glandular breast

5.8   In diagnostic radiography

A   impurities in the tube vacuum increase the efficiency of the tube
B   about half of the electrical energy is converted into X-ray energy
C   the anode stem is lubricated by the oil in the tube housing
D   the efficiency of production of X-rays is higher at higher tube kV
E   focal spot size increases with tube current

5.9   X-ray film

A   emulsion, consists of silver halide suspended in polyester
B   base, is about 0.15 mm thick and is usually tinted blue
C   requires pure silver bromide crystals in the emulsion
D   is usually single sided in mammography
E   is double sided when used in a laser imager

5.10   Regarding modulation transfer function

A   MTF is a continuous function
B   the MTF is plotted as a function of X-ray frequency
C   system MTF is the sum of the MTFs of individual components
D   MTF is 60-75% at zero spatial frequency
E   MTF is a measure of the contrast reduction in objects with small detail

5.11   Regarding computed tomography

A   only axial sections can be scanned
B   CT machines are used for radiotherapy simulation
C   arrays of thallium doped caesium iodide can be used for detection
D   contrast resolution and spatial resolution are unrelated
E   a 4th generation rotate-stationary system uses a 360 degree array of
     stationary detectors

5.12   Regarding patient dose in X-ray imaging

A   in CT, slices adjacent to the scan slice are exposed to stray radiation
B   higher dose increases quantum noise
C   a large focal spot minimizes dose
D   dose is decreased by use of filters to remove low energy X-rays
E   dose is always decreased in magnification radiography

5.13 In digital radiography, the following data manipulation is possible

A background subtraction
B contrast enhancement
C image subtraction of dual energy images
D edge enhancement
E elimination of scatter

5.14 In diagnostic ultrasound

A a piezoelectric crystal is optimally operated at the Curie temperature
B a pulsed electric field causes a change in the shape of the crystal
C improved crystal dampening improves the reception of echoes
D at the resonant frequency, the wavelength is twice the thickness of the crystal
E changing the frequency of ultrasound, usually necessitates changing the transducer

5.15 Regarding ultrasound image quality

A image broadening, caused by finite beam width, is independent of depth
B velocity difference of ultrasound in examination of the lens and humours of the eye can result in displacement of the retina image towards the transducer
C shadowing behind highly attenuating tissue indicates equipment malfunction
D speckle can be caused by the presence of scattering objects separated by less than the axial resolving distance
E acoustic enhancement posterior to low attenuating tissue is eliminated by correct setting of TGC

5.16 Ultrasound performance checks include measurement of

A beam velocity
B penetration
C registration
D pulse repetition frequency
E dynamic range

5.17 The radio frequency pulse in MRI

A produces a varying magnetic field perpendicular to the static field
B causes the protons to precess at the Larmor frequency
C reduces the overall longitudinal magnetization
D reduces the overall transverse magnetization
E causes some nuclei to align themselves anti-parallel to the static magnetic field

5.18 Regarding spatial location of the MRI signal

A an array of detectors is used to give spatial information about the signal
B a slice selecting gradient field is applied whenever the static field is switched on
C slice thickness is increased by increasing either the slope of the gradient field or the bandwidth of the RF pulses
D nuclei precess in different phases after switching off the phase encoding gradient field
E multi-slice imaging involves overlapping pulse sequences of different frequencies

5.19 A technetium generator

A reaches equilibrium between production and decay at 6 hours
B should be eluted daily
C is usually eluted with pure water
D contains Mo-99 suspended in cellulose
E is hand held

5.20 Regarding gamma camera collimators

A parallel-hole collimation typically absorbs 99.9% of incident gamma rays
B increased septal thickness decreases spatial resolution
C increased hole size increases sensitivity
D sensitivity of collimator is independent of patient-collimator distance
E choice of collimator depends on energy of γ-rays

5.21 In the cervical spine

A the cunieform cartilage may be seen on a soft tissue radiograph
B the height of the anterior and posterior aspects of the vertebral bodies C3-T1 should be equal
C the subchondral synchondrosis of the axis is not present beyond the age of 3 years
D a retrotracheal width of 17 mm is normal in a child
E physiological subluxation of C2 on C3 occurs in 25% of children up to 8 years of age

5.22 Regarding the internal auditory meatus

A the ganglion of the vestibular nerve lies within it
B it transmits the labyrinthine artery
C it transmits the unbranched facial nerve
D the roof is composed of the tegmen tympani
E it is up to 2 cm in length

5.23 Concerning the skull sutures

A the mendosal and lambdoid sutures meet at the asterion
B the saggital and coronal sutures meet at the bregma
C the squamous and lambdoid sutures meet at the pterion
D the coronal suture may be absent
E the metopic suture lies in the frontal bone

5.24 The following are paired

A straight sinus
B cavernous sinus
C sigmoid sinus
D transverse sinus
E basal vein

5.25 On a normal plain abdominal radiograph

A the upper limit of the diameter of the transverse colon is 5.5 cm
B the jejunal diameter may normally exceed 2.5 cm
C it is normal to see a fluid level in the stomach when erect
D a caecal fluid level is present in approximately 20%
E pancreatic calcification may be normal

5.26 The abdominal aorta

A enters the abdomen at T10
B gives rise to the coeliac axis at the level of L3
C has three terminal branches
D has four paired lumbar branches
E bifurcates in front of L4 vertebral body

5.27 The inferior vena cava

A is formed in front of the body of L4
B has two suprarenal veins draining into it
C lies anterior to the left common iliac artery
D receives blood from the right gonadal vein
E lies on the right psoas

5.28 The following branch directly from the subclavian artery

A vertebral artery
B superior intercostal artery
C superior thoracic artery
D acromiothoracic artery
E internal thoracic artery

5.29 The oesophagus

A commences at the level of C4
B receives blood from the inferior thyroid artery
C is approximately 32 cm in length
D deviates to the right in the posterior mediastinum
E lies posterior to the hemiazygous veins

5.30 The trachea

A calcifies more often in men than women
B is about 10 cm in length
C lies posterior to the pulmonary trunk
D is composed of complete fibrocartilaginous rings
E bifurcates behind the sternal angle

5.31 Concerning the carpal bones

A the scaphoid has a distal arterial blood supply
B the capitate articulates with the lunate
C the capitate articulates with only the 2nd and 3rd metacarpals
D all carpal ossification centres have appeared by 8 years of age
E the pisiform is a sesamoid bone

5.32 At birth the following are visible on a plain radiograph

A clavicle
B capitate
C lower femoral ossification centre
D scaphoid
E navicular

5.33 The following form or contribute to a radial/ulnar arterial anastomosis

A anterior interosseous artery
B posterior interosseous artery
C deep palmar arch
D arteria princeps pollicis artery
E superficial palmar arch

5.34 Concerning the veins of the leg

A the anterior tibial vein drains into the popliteal vein
B the profunda femoris vein drains into the great saphenous vein
C the posterior tibial vein drains into the great saphenous vein
D all the veins contain valves
E the short saphenous vein lies superficially

5.35 The male urethra

A receives blood from the pudendal artery
B is split into three anatomical parts
C the seminal colliculus opens into the membranous urethra
D is dilated proximally to form the intrabulbar fossa
E is about 10 cm long

5.36 Concerning the female pelvis

A the bladder is suspended by the median umbilical ligament
B the femoral nerve lies on the iliopsoas muscle
C the round ligament may be seen on CT
D the pudendal canal lies on the medial wall of the ischiorectal fossa
E pectineus passes through the greater sciatic notch

5.37 The axillary artery

A lies inferior to the shoulder joint
B lies posterior to the pectoralis minor
C is medial to the axillary vein
D is closely related to the trunks of the brachial plexus
E extends to the lower edge of teres minor

5.38 Concerning dentition

A the deciduous teeth erupt between 6 and 24 months
B the root is held in position by the peridontal membrane
C there are 12 deciduous incisor teeth
D the central incisors have a unilateral nerve supply
E the upper molars have two roots

5.39 Regarding the gallbladder and bile ducts

A the gallbladder lies partially on the transverse colon
B the gallbladder receives innervation from the vagus
C the fundus is covered by peritoneum
D the common bile duct may measure up to 1 cm in diameter normally
E the gallbladder is supported by a ligament from the inferior surface of the liver

5.40 The following form part of the medial wall of the orbit

A sphenoid bone
B ethmoid bone
C maxilla
D palatine bone
E zygoma

5.41 Regarding T-tube cholangiography

A the tube is normally inserted after exploration of the common bile duct
B it is usually performed by the surgeon
C it is unusual to require a pre-contrast film
D it may cause abdominal pain
E urograffin 370 is a suitable contrast agent

5.42 Concerning cervical myelography

A 10 ml of 300 mg.I/ml of contrast medium is required if contrast is run up from the lumbar region
B the run up is performed with the patient in the lateral decubitus position
C the sequence of radiographs should finish with a supine view
D direct C1/2 puncture is performed with the patient in a lateral position
E special caution should be exercised with chronic schizophrenics

5.43 Regarding superior venacavography

A it is contraindicated in patients with prosthetic heart valves
B the most prominent arm vein should be catheterized
C the catheter should be advanced as close to the subclavian vein as possible
D a left sided injection is satisfactory if superior vena cava obstruction is not suspected
E when bilateral, injection catheters should be linked via a 'Y' connector

5.44 Glucagon

A should be used in preference to buscopan in acromegalics
B dose is 1 mg IV for an adult barium enema
C may cause hypersensitivity reactions in patients with peptic ulceration
D should be used with caution in diabetics
E is contraindicated in thyrotoxicosis

5.45 Regarding sinography

A a control radiograph is mandatory
B the opening of the sinus should be indicated with a radiopaque marker
C if a fistula to the bowel is strongly suspected then dilute barium can be used
D if used, a Foley catheter should be inserted as far into the track as possible
E intermittent screening should be performed during injection of the contrast medium

5.46 Concerning adverse reactions to intravenous iodinated contrast media

A minor reactions occur as frequently as 1:15 administrations
B when used in a patient with congestive cardiac failure mortality maybe as high as 1:500
C there is an 80% recurrence rate after a previous adverse reaction
D a prophylactic regimen combined with a non-ionic agent may reduce the chance of recurrence to less than 1%
E use of a non-ionic agent reduces the chance of a non-fatal reaction by a factor of three to six

5.47 Gadolinium DTPA

A increases signal on a T_1 weighted image
B increases signal on a T_2 weighted image
C can lead to a faster imaging sequence
D is licensed for use as an oral contrast agent
E traverses the intact blood-brain barrier

5.48 The following radiographic centring points are correct

A lateral view of the toes: head of the first metatarsal
B lateral view of the ankle: lateral malleolus
C axial view of the calcaneum: 2.5 cm below the medial malleolus
D 'tunnel' view of knee for intercondylar notch: 2.5 cm below the apex of the patella
E anteroposterior view of the pelvis: upper border of the symphysis pubis

5.49 The zygomatic arch is clearly demonstrated on

A   a lateral skull view
B   a 30 degrees occipitomental facial view
C   a 30 degrees fronto-occipital (Towne's) view
D   a submentovertical skull view
E   an occipitofrontal skull view

5.50 The following radiopharmaceuticals maybe used to assess urine formation and drainage

A ^{99m}Tc DTPA
B ^{99m}Tc Hippuran
C ^{99m}Tc Glucoheptonate
D ^{99m}TDMSA
E ^{99m}Tc MAG-3

5.51 Radionuclide thyroid imaging

A ^{99m}Tc pertechnetate is a useful radiopharmaceutical
B ^{123}I sodium iodide is cheap and readily available
C ^{131}I sodium iodide is satisfactory for routine work
D   a pinhole collimator is used in the detection of ectopic thyroid tissue
E   all thyroid medication should be withdrawn prior to the study

5.52 Concerning barium swallow for motility disorders

A   video or cine facility is mandatory in the upper oesophagus
B   a PA and lateral chest radiograph is a useful adjunct
C   a prone swallow is essential
D   when performed prone the patient should be in the LAO position
E   the oesophagus should be seen to empty completely in the prone position

5.53   Concerning a small bowel enema using a Bilbao-Dotter tube

A   nasal intubation is aided by keeping the patient's neck in the neutral position
B   swallowing of the tube is aided by extending the patient's neck
C   the guide wire is removed when the catheter reaches the pyloric antrum
D   passage from the stomach to the duodenum is encouraged by leaving the patient in the left lateral position
E   water can be swallowed after the barium infusion to maintain its flow to the terminal ileum

5.54   Regarding the instant barium enema

A   it is used to show the extent and severity of colitis
B   it is contraindicated in toxic megacolon
C   it is often useful in Crohns disease
D   a plain film is mandatory
E CO_2 is preferable to air for insufflation

5.55   Regarding the use of a spin-echo sequence in magnetic resonance imaging

A   a TR of greater than 500 msec is considered long
B   a TE of less than 80 msec is considered short
C   if the TR and TE are long then the scan will be T_2 weighted
D   on a T_1 weighted brain scan the grey matter appears grey and the white matter white
E   CSF appears grey on a scan with a long TR and short TE

5.56   Concerning dacrocystography

A   epiphora is the main indication
B   water soluble contrast medium is unsatisfactory
C   subtraction macroradiography is optimal
D   both canaliculi are cannulated
E   the catheter should be secured at least 6 mm inside the duct

5.57 **In ultrasound foetal cardiac anatomy**

A the heart should occupy about 66.6% of the chest cavity
B the moderator band maybe seen in the left ventricle
C the right ventricle lies nearest the anterior chest wall
D both ventricles are of approximately equal size
E on the four chamber view, the flap of the foramen ovale lies in the right atrium

5.58 **Regarding hysterosalpingography**

A a control radiograph should be taken
B urograffin 150 is a suitable contrast medium
C the speculum is withdrawn prior to exposure of radiographs
D a radiograph should be taken prior to the Fallopian tubes outlining with contrast
E buscopan should be given if the tubes fail to 'fill and spill'

5.59 **Concerning intravenous urography**

A if the same amount of iodine is injected the pelvicalyceal systems are opacified better by sodium salts than methylglucamine salts of contrast media
B low osmolar contrast media should be used in infants and small children
C in adults, contrast medium should be injected over about half a minute
D high osmolar contrast media may be used in the elderly
E low osmolar contrast media are excreted slightly earlier than high osmolar media

5.60 **Regarding micturating cystourethrography in infants and children**

A it may be performed under sedation
B an 8F feeding catheter is suitable
C in infants, bladder filling continues until contrast media is seen to track alongside the catheter into the urethra
D removal of the catheter is obligatory before micturition is complete
E a full length KUB radiograph should be taken at the end of the procedure

ANSWERS TO EXAMINATION ONE

The correct answers appear in bold

1.1 B
- A   outside of nucleus
- C   aluminium = -1.5 keV, tungsten = -69.5 keV

1.2 B C D
- A   scatter and attenuation without absorption
- D   but more in a forward direction
- E   1.02 MeV

1.3 B C
- A   J/m²/sec
- B   E = hf (h = Plancks constant)
- C   by definition, in distinction to X-rays
- D   J/sec

1.4 B E
- A   employer
- C   doses likely to exceed 10% of dose limit
- D   defined in local rules which contain systems of work

1.5 C D E
- A   coulombs per kilogram
- B   gray
- D   sieverts

1.6 D E
- A   double emulsion which have different gammas to increase measured range
- B   usually 2-monthly but there is no definite period
- C   however an image of a bone (e.g. rib) or other body part will indicate this
- D   usually caesium-137
- E   because of the filters in the holder

1.7 C E
- A   both A and B are properties utilized in the anode

1.8 A C

B converse
D movement unsharpness
E not related to geometry

1.9 C D

A mesh placed on cassette surface
B just the film
D for name marking after radiograph taken
E low atomic number front and high atomic number back to cassette

1.10 A B C E

C ring artefacts are rare, but can arise if the tube is malaligned in a fixed-rotate scanner; streak artefacts are due to very dense materials that do permit any X-ray transmission
D considerably shorter

1.11 C D

A their main disadvantage is that they cannot be used for this
B synchronization is avoided to prevent 'stroboscopic effect'
D bucky factor = incident radiation/transmitted radiation
E focal distance is from the grid to the convergent point (from which the minimum primary radiation is absorbed)

1.12 A D E

A but resolution is decreased
B multiple needle-like crystals
C electrons from photocathode are accelerated

1.13 A B D E

B acoustic impedance (Z) = density x velocity
$((Z_2 - Z_1) / (Z_2 + Z_1))^2$ x 100 = % of power reflected
C air = 4 x 10^2 kg/m^2/sec
fat = 1.38 x 10^6 kg/m^2/sec
D therefore it is best to scan with beam perpendicular to tissue interface
E by increasing its absorption

1.14 A D E

A homogenous speckled pattern of liver
B this is mirror imaging, which occurs on either side of a strong reflector
C acoustic enhancement occurs behind weakly attenuating structures
D and increasing the PRF
E reverberation artefact

1.15 B C E
    A outer elements before inner ones
    B without the need for sophisticated electronics
    D cannot beam steer with an annular array
    E optimally ¼ λ thick

1.16 C
    A frequency of precession
    B directly proportional
    D radiofrequency

1.17 C E
    A spin-lattice
    D 100-2000 msec
    E longitudinal magnetization cannot be detected above a static field

1.18 A E
    B long TR
    C TE/2 later
    D long TR, short TE

1.19 B D
    A some daily tests
    B e.g. Tc-99m and Co-57
    C flood source

1.20 A B C D
    E unlabelled kits are not radioactive

1.21 A B C E
    D develops from the 2nd and 3rd pharyngeal cartilage

1.22 A B C
    C inside the ligament of Zinn with upper and lower divisions of 5th,
       nasocillary, whereas the trochlear, frontal and lacrimal lie outside
    D passes through the inferior orbital fissure
    E passes through the optic canal

1.23 C E
    A branch of the thyrocervical trunk
    B internal carotid
    D maxillary

1.24 **C D E**
A average 135 ml
B flow rate 500 ml/day

1.25 **A B D**
B also the aortic arch, the left main bronchus and atrium
C mixed with parasympathetic supply from the vugi
D Scatzki B ring represents lower limit of ampulla, A ring the upper, Z line oesophagogastric junction
E 25 cm

1.26 **A B C**
D both do
E R phrenic pierces the diaphragm at T8, the left branches before piercing it

1.27 **A B D E**
B gastrosplenic ligament
C at the hilum
D lienorenal and gastrosplenic ligament
E via pancreaticosplenic nodes

1.28 **B D E**
A the first 2 cm has similar peritoneal relations to the stomach
C superior mesenteric artery

1.29 **A B C D E**

1.30 **A B C D**

1.31 **A B C D E**

1.32 **A B E**
C 4th right costal cartilage
D 5-15 mm

1.33 **A B D**
C navicular
E 1st and 2nd metatarsal

1.34 **A C E**
B there is an S shaped mid carpal joint through which the proximal row articulate with the distal row

1.35 B E
- A at the age of 3 years
- C posterior cruciate arises from the posterior intercondylar region and the anterior cruciate from the anterior intercondylar area attaching to the lateral condyle
- D the larger lateral femoral condyle reduces risk of lateral dislocation

1.36 C D
- A 11 cm, sacral promontory to superior aspect of pubic symphysis
- B 10 cm, tip of coccyx to inferior aspect of pubic symphysis.
- E 128 degrees-adult, 160 degrees-birth

1.37 D
- A connects the atria
- B joins the pulmonary trunk to the aortic arch
- C connects the umbilical vein to the inferior vena cava
- E internal iliac; hence the course of an umbilical artery catheter on AXR

1.38 A B C D E
- B superior and inferior vesical arteries
- C sympathetic supply via the pelvic plexus

1.39 A B D
- B via the inferior thyroid vein to the brachiocephalic
- C 1st and 2nd pharyngeal pouches
- E the isthmus

1.40 A D E
- B malleus is in contact with the tympanic membrane
- C tensor tympani is supplied by the mandibular nerve
- D sensory nerve

1.41 A B D E
- A maximizes soft tissue differentiation
- B causes preferential excretion by the liver
- C total of 6 g taken at 14 h and 3-4 h prior to the examination

1.42 A B C D E
- B to prevent retrograde flow of contrast into the collecting bag
- C to ensure the system is free of air bubbles.
- E the sinus tract is catheterized with a steerable catheter through which a Dormia basket is fed

1.43   **A E**
A   at least 5 days should elapse in order to prevent the injection of contrast into a pool of CSF at the previous puncture site
B   only for very anxious patients
C   it can usually be dispensed with, especially if a narrow gauge (24 SWG) needle is used
D   3 g is the most quoted maximum figure
E   it should be regarded as an inpatient procedure

1.44   **A B D E**
B   evaluation of the venous system following deep vein thrombosis
D   for 4-6 hours, anticipating contrast media induced nausea

1.45   **B C E**
D   this α blocker is the mainstay of treatment for a hypertensive crisis
E   all iodinated contrast media

1.46   **C D**
A   neurotoxic
B   a mixture of sodium and meglumine salts is desirable
C   the non-ionics now in widespread use are still less uncomfortable
D   pure meglumine salts or non-ionic contrast media should be used for venography
E   only non-ionic agents

1.47   **D E**
A   200-250%
B   intermediate density (130-150%)
C   not if any possibility of aspiration
D   some ionic contrast may be absorbed through gastrointestinal mucosa
E   very poor mucosal coating

1.48   **A B C D**
E   occipitofrontal without angulation

1.49   **A B D**
C   patient prone and turned 45 degrees RAO
E   oblique views of the lumbar spine demonstrate the pars interarticularis on the side to which the patient is turned

1.50   **A D E**
B   550-1200 MBq
D   to prevent uptake by normal choroid plexus, thyroid and salivary glands
E   because of their blood flow

1.51 A B D E
   A for the demonstration of pre and post renal causes
   B blood supply, parenchymal damage and trauma to the collecting
      system
   C the spatial resolution is insufficient to detect small tumours
   D by either introducing isotope into the bladder directly or following a
      standard renal study
   E ^{123}I Hippuran or ^{99m}Tc DTPA or ^{99m}Tc MAG3 may be used to demon-
      strate renal artery stenosis

1.52 A B C D
   C to ascertain if there is normal gland tissue beyond it
   E this is a contraindication

1.53 B E
   A pass nasogastric tube into pouch and take a chest radiograph
   B if a fistula from the bronchial tree exists, as it usually does, then there
      will be air in the fundus and the extent can be measured
   C if table upright and infant horizontal and face down then a shoot
      through lateral can be performed
   D barium may be aspirated via the larynx and cause diagnostic difficul-
      ties
   E a true AP and lateral radiograph show a typical impression at aortic
      arch level

1.54 A C D E
   B insulin dependent diabetics should be first on a morning list, omit
      morning dose, take a reduced dose of insulin after the examination
   C they are admitted in many centres in order to monitor fluid balance
   D desacetylbisacodyl from picosulphate and magnesium citrate from
      magnesium oxide and citric acid
   E at least 45 minutes to allow reabsorbtion of retained fluid thus improv-
      ing mucosal coating

1.55 B D
   A high density barium in the bowel will cause streak artefact
   B so that the stomach is completely outlined with oral contrast
   C a full bladder is required to elevate small bowel loops out of the pelvis
   D the last glass should be saved for about 5 minutes prior to the scan in
      order to outline the duodenal loop

1.56 A C D E
   B high intensity on T1
   D due to fat suppression on the Short Tau Inversion Recovery (STIR)
      sequence

1.57   B C

A   the internal os. This is because the trigone of the bladder is fixed to the cervix and does not change position as the bladder fills
D   this may be done by seeing the vessels entering laterally
E   the obturator internus may be. Levator ani's attachment to the vaginal vault marks the lower limit of the ovarian position

1.58   B D

A   45 degrees
C   as it travels obliquely through the liver, this would give an oblique rather than true transverse section
D   in this case abdominal circumference should be measured above the level of the kidneys and below the level of the heart pulsation
E   with two branches of portal vein and ductus venosus

1.59   D

B   no indication in patients with uncomplicated epididymoorchitis
C   in adult women a clinically relevant abnormality is seldom demon-strated
D   an alternative modality should be used
E   urographic contrast can block the uptake of therapeutic and diagnostic radioisotopes of iodine

1.60   A D

B   this is one of the main indications for the procedure
C   the ureter is catheterized at cystoscopy, normally performed by a urologist
D   if possible
E   urograffin 150, so that small filling defects are not obscured by a high concentration of contrast

ANSWERS TO EXAMINATION TWO

The correct answers appear in bold

2.1   ALL FALSE
    B   expressed as Bq/mol or Bq/kg
    C   it is a constant
    D   from the nucleus
    E   helium nucleus

2.2   **A C E**
    B   not EM radiation
    C   infra-red = 10^{-4} to 10^{-6} m, visible light = 5×10^{-7} m
    D   inversely proportional

2.3   **A C**
    B   it is the thermoluminescent material that fluoresces, usually lithium fluoride or calcium sulphate
    D   there is no image formation

2.4   **A B**
    C   500 mSv, 50 mSv is the dose limit for a member of the public
    D   13 mSv
    E   this is the recommendation of the ICRP in 1990 but has not been introduced into UK legislation

2.5   **B E**
    B   prior to MRI
    C   does not affect management
    D   maybe required if IUCD not seen on ultrasound
    E   ultrasound and plain abdominal X-ray may be preferred in young patients

2.6   **A C D**
    B   natural 87% (radon 47% of total background) artificial 13% (medical 12% of total background) i.e. medical is majority of man made background radiation
    C   approximately 1.3 mSv from disintegrations of radon, polonium, bismuth and lead
    D   radon gas builds up in poorly ventilated and double glazed buildings
    E   Cornwall and Scotland

2.7　A B C
A　proportional to kV^2
B　intensity may be defined as the product of the number of photons in the beam and energy of each photon, so it also increases with mA

2.8　E
A　materials tend to be transparent to their own characteristic radiation
B　half value layer = $0.693/\mu$
C　low energy radiation retained in beam
D　in compound Al/Cu filter the aluminium absorbs the characteristic radiation of copper and lies nearest the patient
E　IRR 85 Guidance notes (ICRP 33 1982)

2.9　A B D
A　speed is the reciprocal of the exposure required for a density of 1.0 above base plus fog
C　fog increases with decreasing pH

2.10　B E
A　not possible
B　but beyond a field of 30 cm diameter scatter production plateaus
C　presence of air gap reduces scatter
D　decreased

2.11　A C
B　vidicon camera decreases contrast, TV display increases contrast depending on the camera tube and monitor settings
D　fast film/screen-3 μGy, Cine-100-150 nGy/frame
E　used to split image

2.12　C D
B　also magnetic disc, magnetic tape
C　use of narrow window width
D　use of window level and width
E　4096 shades in 16-bit equipment

2.13　B
A　xenon or xenon/krypton to increase X-ray absorbtion
C　to harden beam
D　256^2, 512^2 or 1024^2
E　CT number represents comparison between linear absortion coefficient of a pixel and that of water (so water is 0)

2.14 **A B C D E**
  B shorter pulse length, therefore increased axial resolution
  C less than half the object separation

2.15 **D**
  A Doppler shift equation
  B higher frequency transducer
  C 2D real time image plus pulsed wave doppler
  D Nyquist frequency is the maximum frequency of the Doppler shift that can be detected unambiguously
  E half the pulse repetition frequency. Sampling theory dictates that the sampling frequency (PRF) should be greater than or equal to half the observed frequency (DS)

2.16 **ALL FALSE**
  A liquid Helium: 4K
  B 2 Tesla
  C attracted to magnet
  D iron cage and copper wire cage (Faraday cage)
  E RF field

2.17 **B C**
  A TE/2
  B allows T2 versus T2* effects to be measured
  D short TE
  E start of sequence to start of next sequence

2.18 **A B C D**
  B so that it is eliminated quickly thereby reducing dose
  C in practice 50-300 KeV
  D 100% of desired isotope and no contaminants of other isotopes of that element

2.19 **ALL FALSE**
  A a single large crystal is used
  B sodium iodide doped with thallium
  C the crystal lies between the collimator and the PMTs
  D hexaganol or circular
  E it generates the Z energy signal. The position decoding matrix generates the X and Y coordinates

2.20 C
A   511 keV produced by the positron annilation
B   very short: minutes - hours
D   multiple detectors for higher sensitivity
E   positrons have high kinetic energy, so high dose

2.21 C D E
A   external carotid artery
B   external carotid artery. Both the ascending pharyngeal via foramen
     lacerum and the occipital via jugular foramen have meningeal supply

2.22 B
A   middle meningeal artery: foramen spinosum
C   maxillary nerve: foramen rotundum
D   palatine foramen: palatine vessels
E   glossopharyngeal nerve: jugular foramen

2.23 A C E
B   in about 4% of adults
D   superior orbital fissure, though a branch pterygoid plexus may pass
     through inferior orbital fissure

2.24 A B D E

2.25 B C D
C   greater and lesser omentum
E   left vagus

2.26 A B C D
A   to anastomose with SMV behind neck of pancreas
E   receives blood from the splenic artery

2.27 A C D
B   posterior
D   thus hypertrophy can cause medial deviation
E   narrowed at the pelviureteric junction, pelvic brim and ureterovesical
     junction

2.28 A B C
D   right hepatic artery in the majority

2.29 D E
A   anterior sinus
B   T4
C   both are anterior

2.30 D
- A opposite way around
- B 3rd intercostal space
- C 2.5 cm
- D conus arteriosus = infundibulum
- E 4th and 5th intercostal spaces

2.31 A
- B T5 left brachiocephalic crosses at T4 anterior to the artery
- C T4-5, as low as T6 on deep inspiration
- D loops around the right main bronchus, not present at this level

2.32 A C D

2.33 B C E

2.34 A C D
- A the antero-inferior 1/3
- B secondary cartilaginous joint
- E eight

2.35 B C
- A axillary artery
- D other way around
- E superior intercostal artery is a branch of the costocervical trunk

2.36 A B E
- A the cruciate ligaments
- C converse is true

2.37 C E
- A 5 and 12 weeks
- B 8th week
- D two arteries and one vein

2.38 A B C
- B cistern relates to splenium above, vermis below, and tent and falx posteriorly
- D foramen of Munro
- E foramen of Magendie

2.39 C D E
- A superior medullary velum spans between them
- B pons
- E and via the foramina of Lushka into the pontine cistern

2.40   A B E
B   valve of Rosenmuller
C   3 cm

2.41   E
B   T2 weighting
C   unlike the spin echo the gradient echo sequence does not cancel field inhomogeneity
D   5-15 degrees

2.42   A C E
A   to exclude a thoracic aortic aneurysm
B   undercouch, to reduce radiation dose to the endoscopist
D   2-5 ml
E   prone or prone oblique to prevent aspiration

2.43   A B E
A   easier usually than alternative lateral decubitus
C   the needle should be rotated to prevent the bevel lying across the dura and resulting in an extra dural injection
D   only in direct cervical puncture and if there is uncertainty about the position of the needle
E   too rapid injection causes unwanted turbulence in the CSF

2.44   ALL FALSE
A   usually because the ankle tourniquet has not been properly applied
B   the needle should not be removed
C   approximately 250 mg iodine/ml, which is equivalent 50 ml of 300 mg iodine/ml solution diluted with 10 ml of saline
D   the amount is variable due to differing venous capacities of limbs. It should be determined by fluoroscopy
E   hand injection using extension tubing so that venous extravasation maybe detected

2.45   C D
A   one of its advantages is that it can be performed as an outpatient
B   contrast maybe delivered through a wide bore cannula in the ante-cubital fossa
D   by preventing bowel movement artefacts
E   this a technique used to re-register the mask in order to compensate for minor degrees of patient movement

2.46 B
- A 640 mmol/kg at 37°C
- B ionic dimer
- C non-ionic dimer
- D even up to concentrations of 400 mg/ml iotrolan is, but it is viscous
- E mostly non-ionic, except ioxaglate

2.47 A B C D
- A bowel 'pseudotumour' is a common pitfall in abdominal CT
- B also sometimes in pelvic scanning
- C use of a vaginal tampon exploits this
- D usual vascular supply of metastases is from hepatic artery that enhances before the portal circulation
- E delay to allow dilution and mixture in CSF

2.48 A B D E

2.49 A C
- A quiet respiration, to help blur out the ribs
- B arrested respiration
- C during inspiration
- D a double exposure technique is used. An exposure is made on full inspiration and another during full expiration on the same film

2.50 C D E
- A ^{99m}Tc pyrophosphate
- B imaging should be performed 1-3 days after the acute event
- D less than 20% may be positive
- E it is more sensitive, improves localisation of the site of infarction and can be used to estimate the mass of infarcted tissue

2.51 B C D E
- A patients should be well hydrated and empty their bladders prior to scanning
- B linked to a phosphate analogue, e.g. methylene diphosphonate

2.52 C

A this makes the duct more difficult to cannulate. The mucosa should be dried with a swab, the gland may be massaged to produce a bead of saliva

B about 1 cm. Up to the point when resistance is felt as the duct penetrates buccinator

C more in a diseased gland

D up to 2 ml may be injected but acinar filling can occur before pain arises, and the patient should not speak. A prearranged signal is required

E this interferes with radiography. Should be taped to contralateral side

2.53 E

A at least 6 hours of fasting

B rolled supine to allow barium to wash over the gastro-oesophageal junction

C LAO position used for lesser curve

D slightly elevated helps to empty barium from the apex of the cap into the second part of the duodenum and fill the duodenal cap with air

E with a cup and spill fundus

2.54 B

A prone

B because the valve lies on the medial posterolateral wall

C prone

D should not be used unless absolutely necessary

E muscle relaxants allow greater colonic distension and haustra are less pronounced

2.55 C E

A as CT has greater contrast resolution

B it may show intraspinal invasion of adjacent tumour and may provide valuable information about pathology above the level of a block on a conventional myelogram

C to improve spatial resolution

E or disc prolapse

2.56 D E

A low intensity

B this is a great advantage of MRI

C inability to demonstrate calcification is a limitation of MRI

D the appearance changes with changes in the chemical composition of the haematoma. Initially it may have the same signal as brain

E because the supportive equipment is still often incompatible with use in an MR scanner and the duration of the scan may be unacceptable

2.57 **B D**

    A the gestational sac must be seen within the uterus

    C within it

    E 7-12 weeks

2.58 **D**

    A it is however advisable

    B although a small amount of urine may help with orientation

    C the converse is true

    D this is a useful technique for anxious patients

    E usually twice a day or is necessary if the condom ruptures

2.59 **C D**

    A George, C.D. *et al.*, *BJR*, 66, 17-19

    B in order to reduce the possibility of vomiting

    C and in infants and patients with myeloma and renal failure. Though it does not lead to any improvement in the image and is not to be recommended generally (Bell, K.E. *et al.*, *Clin Rad*, 36, 311-314)

    D paraproteins may precipitate in the tubules causing acute renal failure, an alternative modality should be used if possible

    E the bladder should be emptied prior to the procedure in order that the contrast media is not overly diluted by urine

2.60 **A**

    A UTI should be treated prior to the procedure

    B 5-10 ml for the pelvicalyceal system and less for the ureter

    C it should be slowly withdrawn while contrast is injected to delineate the ureter

    D the contrast medium should be aspirated and a radiograph taken to demonstrate the residuum and any hold up

    E this usually means too much contrast has been injected and pyelosinus backflow has occurred

ANSWERS TO EXAMINATION THREE

The correct answers appear in bold

3.1 **A**
B physical methods
D exponential process and therefore never reaches zero
E rate of decay or number of disintegrations per second (Becquerels)

3.2 **A B**
B because compared with the focal distance the focal spot behaves as a point source
D units are keV/micron, it determines the quality factor

3.3 **A B C D**
B up to 10 times greater. This has important implications for staff radiation protection e.g. when screening using an over-couch tube
C up to approximately 1 MeV
D number of electrons per gram influences level of Compton scatter
E less scatter but more in a forward direction

3.4 **A B C**
B IRR 88 (POPUMET) - protection of persons undergoing medical examination or treatment
C but must be under the direction of an ARSAC licence holder
D granted to consultant radiologist who clinically directs work
E NHS hospitals with Trust status are not exempt

3.5 **B D**
A normally attached to local medical physics department
C no, consultant radiologist is clinically directing (IRR 88)
D IRR 88
E physically and clinically directing

3.6 **B C E**
C prior to bone marrow transplantation
D radiation once used to treat this condition
E others include vascular changes, lens opacification and stem cell ablation

3.7 **A D**
B anode side
C converse is true
D arises from regions outside of focal spot
E up to 15-20 %.

3.8   **A C**
B   converse
C   greatest at short exposures
D   converse
E   smaller anode angle has higher rating

3.9   **A C**

3.10   **B E**
A $\log_{10} I_0 / I_T$ I_0 = incident, I_T = transmitted
B   contrast = $density_2$ - $density_1$
C   there is a finite density due to base and fog (0.15)
D   0.25 to 2.5
E   this is the value of using a logarithmic scale

3.11   **A B D E**
C   speed is the reciprocal of exposure that gives unit density above base plus fog
D   it has smaller crystals
E   a fast film generally has a wide range of, and larger crystal size giving a small gamma

3.12   **D E**
A   0.5-1 mm
B   superior at low contrast
C   inversely proportional
D   at the detector, noise is determined by the number of photons absorbed (detected)

3.13   **B D**
A   between normal to slice and detector axis
B   i.e. the section thickness is inversely proportional to the amplitude of tube movement
C   thin slice and poor contrast
D   around the fulcrum
E   longer

3.14   **B E**
A   TGC compensates for the stronger attenuation of echoes from deeper than superficial structures
C   regulates amplification of echoes from all depths
D   echoes with amplitude below a certain threshold are rejected
E   echoes amplified from a gated portion of the TGC slope

3.15 A B C E

D during microcavitation ionization can occur but this has not been demonstrated with diagnostic ultrasound

3.16 A D

3.17 B D E

A to 37% of its original value
C as moments move out of phase
D hence T2* versus T2 weighting

3.18 B

A low degree
C decreases T2
D decrease T1 and T2
E vice versa

3.19 A B

A as it is in its metastable state
C 140 keV
D physical half life
E Tc-99

3.20 D

A crystal is hygroscopic
B maximum count rate
C 2×10^4 counts per second
D not just removal of scatter, they help detector system ascribe a point of origin to the detected photons
E analogue-to-digital converter required

3.21 B

A occipital bone
C petrous bone
D greater wing of sphenoid
E greater wing of sphenoid

3.22 A B D E

D and falx
E also: habenular commisure; choroid plexus; arachnoid granulations; basal ganglia; dentate nucleus; carotid artery and lens of eye

3.23 A D

D superficial to the external carotid

3.24 **D E**
   A L3
   B C7
   C T7 and 7th intercostal space

3.25 **C D E**
   A L1/2
   B renal vein
   C relations at renal hilum, from anterior to posterior-vein artery, pelvis artery

3.26 **A C E**
   B common hepatic, left gastric and splenic arteries
   D 2 cm
   E via the left gastric artery

3.27 **C D E**
   A 2% of body weight (1.5 kg)
   B four: falciform ligament, coronary ligament, right and left triangular ligaments

3.28 **A B C**
   C other anterior division branches are inf. gluteal, obturator, uterine, inferior and superiorvesical (posterior division iliolumbar, sup. gluteal and lat. sacral)
   D aorta
   E ileocolic artery

3.29 **D**
   A 38-45 cm
   B posterior at this level
   C T12
   D and then forwards in front of the subclavian artery
   E left brachiocephalic vein

3.30 **B C E**
   A becomes the coronary sinus
   D remnant of the left superior vena cava
   E small veins draining much of cardiac wall directly into heart chambers

3.31 **B C**
   D medial segment middle lobe
   E left upper lobe bronchus

3.32 **A B**
   C   the facets of the 10th, 11th, and 12th are single
   D   three primary and five secondary centres
   E   upwards, useful when identifying cervical ribs

3.33 **A C E**
   A   capitellum
   B   radial head
   C   internal epicondyle
   D   trochlear
   E   olecranon, external epicondyle

3.34 **A D E**
   B   <23 mm in males and <21.5 mm in females
   C   lateral to the cuboid
   D   posterior tibiotalar part
   E   calcaneofibular part

3.35 **B D E**
   A   arises laterally then spirals deep to adductor longus
   B   along with deep and superficial external pudendal, and superficial
       circumflex iliac
   D   along with lateral circumflex femoral and four perforating branches

3.36 **A B C D E**
   E   rotator cuff: subscapularis, infraspinatus, supraspinatus and teres minor

3.37 **A B C D**
   E   both

3.38 **A D**
   B   but pubocervical, lateral cervical and uterosacral ligaments do support
   D   which anastomoses with the uterine artery within the broad ligament
   E   10-12 cm long, 1 cm wide

3.39 **A B E**
   A   at hiatus semilunaris anterior to middle ethmoid and maxillary
       posteriorly
   C   middle meatus
   D   inferior meatus
   E   forming the torus tubarius

3.40   B C D E
A except stylopharynx
E down to cricopharyngeus

3.41   A B E
C 20 degrees obliquely to the right, to project the common duct clear of
   the vertebral column
D injection should be fractionated and radiographs exposed simultane-
   ously

3.42   B C D E
A 70-75 kV
D it is very important to have the positioning clear in your mind

3.43   A C
A non-ionic agents cause less damage to the vascular endothelium, lower
   the incidence of thrombus formation and cause less discomfort
B exposures are made when calf veins are maximally filled
C thrombi may originate in foot veins
D it is performed to demonstrate the proximal segment of the deep
   femoral vein
E ambulation or exercise is important to discourage thrombus formation

3.44   A B D E
E also tachycardia it induces may precipitate angina

3.45   D E
A there is a delay (depending on the area of the body to be imaged and
   the cardiac output) to allow contrast to circulate before image acquisi-
   tion
B conventional contrast media can be administered through a central
   venous catheter
C it is valuable in diagnosis of PE
D put patients with renal impairment should be examined intra-arterially
E particularly valuable for investigation of pulmonary vascular anoma-
   lies

3.46   B D
A more dilution because of the osmotic diuresis
C ionic agents do. Special care must be taken to regularly flush catheters
   and exclude blood clot from syringes during angiography
D Ansell G., *Prescribers Journal*, 33-2, 82-88
E safety in pregnancy not established

3.47 A B
 B free gadolinium is toxic
 C alters behaviour of tissues surrounding contrast
 D usually 0.1 mmol/kg maybe 0.2 mmol/kg
 E excretion is via the kidneys

3.48 A B D E
 C remote from the film

3.49 A B C E
 D 15 degrees of caudal angulation
 E on an AP oblique the foramina nearest the tube are demonstrated

3.50 A B D E
 A this still the most commonly used
 B it is this property that makes it valuable for imaging
 C the patient should be fasted for 4 hours to reduce splanchnic blood
    flow and have all cardiac medication, particularly β-blockers, stopped
 D using exercise or pharmacologically
 E before and at least 3 days after the angioplasty

3.51 A B C D E
 A this property is employed in the detection of a Meckels diverticulum
 E the lacrimal glands do take up a small amount of pertechetate but
    dacroscintigraphy is performed by instilling pertechnetate solution
    directly into the lacrimal apparatus

3.52 B C E
 A much more difficult to perform
 B a bead of saliva is seen at the orifice
 C a diseased gland may become insensitive to distension
 D no significant advantage
 E glottic oedema due to allergic reaction to iodine

3.53 A B C D E
 A a long tube is used and barium injected in once the bowel is decom-
    pressed
 B alternatively Silk tube
 C if an adept intubation is performed, and barium is injected by hand
 D rate of flow of intestinal contents is slowed by a full caecum

3.54 A B D
 B to assess retro-rectal space
 C RAO
 E supine

3.55   B D
    A but a full discussion with the parents always is
    B wearing a protective gown
    C malignant disease
    D because of the lack of intra-abdominal and pelvic fat
    E under sedation if possible as general anaesthesia may cause atelectasis and therefore artefacts

3.56   D E
    B along the direction of the beam
    C between two leading edges

3.57   B C E
    A head circumference is preferable for breech or transverse lie
    B because near field resolution is poor
    C and it should not merge with the thigh skin line
    D stripe is discontinuous at the cavum septum pellucidum
    E if correctly performed, BPD used more routinely

3.58   A C D E
    A to enhance soft tissue detail
    B a control radiograph should always be performed just prior to the examination
    C and will tend to swallow more air, thus obscuring the kidneys
    E if the kidneys are obscured by gas or faeces then the need for tomography can be determined

3.59   A B C D E
    A if IV urography has been unsatisfactory
    B and antibiotic prophylaxis should be given routinely
    C very little contrast medium is absorbed systemically, so that hypersensitivity to contrast is only a relative contraindication
    D the bladder must be uncomfortably full if performed following IV urography, but this technique is little used because of the limited information it provides
    E contrast media maybe already in the ureters if performed following IV urography

3.60   ALL FALSE
    A Knuttsons penile clamp or Foley catheter
    B the Foley balloon is partially inflated in the fossa navicularis
    C Urograffin 290
    D micturating cystography should be performed to distend the posterior urethra and sometimes prostatic ducts
    E each side with the leg abducted and the knee flexed

ANSWERS TO EXAMINATION FOUR

The correct answers appear in bold

4.1   C
    A lower end
    B characteristic radiation in association with a photoelectron and a
       positive ion
    D proportional to Z^3
    E bound electrons, in biological tissues from the K shell

4.2   B C
    A exponential process
    B also increases with atomic number and number of electrons per gram
    D attenuation = absorption + scatter
    E 30 mm

4.3   A B C D E
    B stochastic effects have no threshold level, hence importance of
       ALARA principle
    E it is usually assumed that all radiation damage is harmful, although
       stochastic effects are responsible for mutation and evolution

4.4   E
    A workers who receives less than 30% of an annual dose limit can be
       classified but if 30% is exceeded they must be classified
    B average annual dose in North West Regional Health Authority in 1986
       was 0.31 mSv
    C 50 years
    D incumbent on employer to monitor environment and a representative
       sample of staff only

4.5   A D
    B attached below tube
    C estimated by relating incident dose from existing tables
    D female gonad dose more difficult
    E must be three times expected dose for fluoroscopy (Table 1, Guidance
       note PM 77, Regulation 33 of IRR 85)

4.6   C D E
    A the prime responsibility lies with the clinician
    B it is best to ask the patient
    C NRPB
    D NRPB

4.7   A B C
   A   high energy cut off increases with kVp
   B   hardens or, increases the average energy per photon in, the beam
   C   three phase supply gives an average kVp higher than single phase

4.8   C
   C   prevents light diffusion through phosphor
   D   light from upper screen sensitizes lower emulsion (screen unsharpness)
       and there is imperfect overlapping of the images (paralax unsharpness)

4.9   C E
   A   most screens are rare earth now
   B   many crystals packed together
   C   ratio of exposure required without screen to that with screen
   D   e.g. gadolinium oxysulphide, lanthanum oxybromide and calcium
       tungstate
   E   increases efficiency of absorbtion by photoelectric effect

4.10   A D E
   A   this occurs in the solarization portion of the curve
   B   the straight line portion of the curve
   C   logarithmic scale
   D   shifts to the left and is steeper
   E   base plus fog

4.11   C
   A   -1000
   B   centre of range
   D   decrease in density
   E   eight-fold increase: dose α (resolution)^3

4.12   B E
   A   some primary rays removed
   B   increased exposure required
   C   separated by solid of low atomic number
   D   height of strips to separation

4.13   A E
   A   by definition
   C   this occurs with transverse waves, sound waves are longitudinal
   C   1540 m/sec
   D   mW/cm^2. Relative intensity is measured in decibels
   E   when considering potential tissue damage

4.14 A D
A   transmits for about 1/1000th of the time it receives
B   number of ultrasound pulses in 1 second
C   range of frequencies is called the bandwidth
E   shorter pulse duration has a greater bandwidth

4.15 A B C
A   longitudinal cannot be measured above static field
D   decreases
E   10-200 MHz approximately

4.16 A C D
B   reduces TR and imaging time
D   their large magnetic moment increases local field fluctuations
E   high contrast

4.17 A B C E
A   in large blood vessels running perpendicular to the static field
B   some are magnetically programmed, also the leads can act as antennae
    in time varying RF fields. Warning notices are put at the 5G line

4.18 B
A   crystal performance
C   sensitivity increases at the expense of spatial resolution
D   10 mm
E   line source phantom

4.19 D
A   post-scan
B   varying arrival times
C   cardiac studies - highest count rate
E   1 frame/sec during vascular perfusion

4.20 B C
A   inferior
C   decreased patient-camera distance
D   lower

4.21 A B C
B   posterior part with the vomer, anterior part is cartilagenous
E   middle meatus

4.22 A C D
A thoracic and lumbar below
D Moore K.L., *Clinically Orientated Anatomy* (third edition), Williams and Wilkins, London, 1992
E lower intercostal or left lumbar artery

4.23 B D
A superior oblique
C chorda tympani
E pons at the cerebellopontine angle

4.24 B C E
A the oculomotor, trochlear, ophthalmic, and maxillary. The abducent nerve lies medially
B lateral wall
C via foramen ovale, or if present foramen vesalius
D internal carotid artery

4.25 A C D
B three: inferior phrenic-superior adrenal; aorta-middle adrenal; renal-inferior adrenal arteries
E triangular. The left gland is crescentic

4.26 A B D
A IVC is posterior to the foramen, caudate lobe superior and 1st part of duodenum is inferior
C anterior to foramen with the hepatic artery and portal vein

4.27 B C D E
D superior mesenteric may supply all of the right lobe in 10% of people

4.28 A D E
C usually about 1.5 m

4.29 B C D
A 9-16 mm
B and anterior to the right bronchus

4.30 A B D E
D all but the first intercostal eventually drain via the azygous

4.31 A D E
A in approximately 90%, also sinoatrial node in around 50%
B left
C left

4.32 A B C

C anteriorly, the proximal oesophagus may be indented by a venous plexus

E aortic knuckle

4.33 B E

A axis to occiput

C extension of the posterior longitudinal ligament

D connects the dens to the basiocciput

4.34 A B C E

A superiorly ingiunal ligament and medial border of adductor longus

D ASIS and pubic tubercle

4.35 A B D

C superior orbital fissure

E jugular foramen (pars nervosum)

4.36 A B

A sympathetic supply

C left renal vein, derived from part of the subcardinal vein

D aorta

4.37 C D E

A 16 mm

B dorsally

E dorsum sellae is projected over the foramen magnum if correctly angled

4.38 C D

A four: capsular, lateral, sphenomandibular and stylomandibular

B anterior

E both do

4.39 A E

B left lobe

C lateral

D caudate lobe drains directly into the IVC

4.40 A B D

E ischium

4.41 A B C

C also normally there should not be excess retrograde filling of hepatic ducts

4.42 A C E
  B patient on their side
  D 10-15 degrees is usually sufficient

4.43 A E
  B should not be performed unless the epiphyses have fused
  C Lea-Thomas drill tip needle
  D greater trochanter
  E external and common iliac veins in the prone position

4.44 A C D
  B 20 mg
  D may cause temporary loss of accommodation and affect ability to drive
  E it is an antimuscarinic, a quaternary ammonium compound

4.45 B D E
  C a lower concentration of iodine in the contrast medium is required
  D as long as it is given slowly
  E prolonged data acquisition is performed after injection into the splenic or superior mesenteric arteries

4.46 A B
  C gastrografin is used to treat this
  D barium preferable
  E barium should be used with caution in children with cystic fibrosis because of the risk of inspissation

4.47 B C
  A paramagnetic
  B remarkably low side effect profile
  C in epileptics or patients with brain tumours
  D now licensed for children and whole body use
  E insufficient data at present to establish safety

4.48 A B D
  C 2.5 cm distal to the line joining the epicondyles of the humerus
  E 2.5 cm from the sternal end of the clavicle

4.49 A C E
  B increased to 350 cm plus the use of a grid
  D contrast is reduced

4.50 A C D E
    A delivered as an aerosol
    B during deep inspiration
    D it may result in microemboli to the brain
    E if it is normal

4.51 A C D E
    B decreased uptake over the pacemaker site
    E due to dribbling on to the feet during micturition

4.52 A C E
    B water soluble first

4.53 B
    A suspected small intestinal perforation
    B after negative upper and lower GI investigation
    D jejunal biopsy

4.54 A C
    A cleansing water enemas are difficult to perform
    B a catheter with a flange which adheres or is held by the patient, or a
        Foley catheter with 10 ml of air in the balloon
    C or peristalsis causes continual emptying
    D right side to move barium into ascending colon
    E when erect the colon almost always empties

4.55 A D E
    A it is not known to be safe during the first trimester
    B only if they have been shown to be metallic on a plain radiograph
    C only the older variety
    D they may not fit in the scanner
    E the patient must be removed from the room in the event of a cardiac
        arrest

4.56 C D
    A fasted to distend the gallbladder
    B subcostally
    C Platt, J.F. *et al.*, *AJR*, 151-2, 317-319
    E either stays the same or reduces

4.57 B D E
    C not visible in the normal fetus
    D the lateral border of the anterior horn and the insula both lie
        anterolaterally and can both be prominent

4.58   A C E

B   increased. Patients with renal failure require twice the standard amount

D   it is dependent on GFR, sodium and water reabsorption from the proximal tubule, peak plasma contrast concentration and therefore renal blood flow

E   apparent differences in nephrographic density may also be due to rotation of a kidney difference in renal size

4.59   B C D E

A   Foley catheters should not be used because if incorrectly placed in the bladder neck or distal urethra , the bladder may rupture as it is maximally distended with contrast

B   it may be diluted with saline however

4.60   A B C

A   usually only performed if there has been some operative difficulty

D   opiates should be avoided because they can cause tubal spasm

E   the radiologist should be capable of cannulating and inspecting the cervix

ANSWERS TO EXAMINATION FIVE

The correct answers appear in bold

5.1 A D E
A Z = atomic number = 15
B A = mass number = 32
C protons

5.2 ALL FALSE
A slightly more
B interrupted by absorption edges
C used to produce an almost monochromatic beam (K edge molybdenum filter)
D 33 keV, typical X-ray beams have a high proportion of photons at or just above this energy
E this happens when the mean energy of the beam is just below the K edge of the material of higher atomic number

5.3 A E
B discrete energy spectrum
C lower probability of interaction and RBE is also less
D inversely proportional
E as in PET

5.4 B C D E
A this is the effective dose
B ICRP 60
E quality factor of neutrons >20 MeV = 5, alpha particles = 20

5.5 A E
A In North West RHA in 1986 doses were as follows:

mSv	% of total
>15	0.2
10-15	0.2
5-10	2.2
1-5	7.9
<1	89.5

C cardiologists = 1.3 mSv, radiologists = 0.57 mSv, radiographers = 0.36 mSv
D no dose limits for patients whilst undergoing examination

5.6   A E
A   ideally
B   0.25-0.5 mm
C   staff should never be in the primary beam
D   used for protection against transmitted beam
E   0.25 mm = 8.6% , 0.35 mm = 4.6%

5.7   C E
D   every 3 years

5.8   D E
B   99% of energy converted into heat
C   silver. Oil helps cool the housing, surrounding the tube
D   kV   Heat %   X-rays
    60   99.5   0.5
    200   99.0   1.0
    4000   60.0   40
E   focal spot blooming

5.9   B D
A   polyester forms base
C   requires impurities to form sensitivity speck
D   emulsion adjacent to screen on side remote from breast
E   single sided

5.10   A E
A   MTF of 1 means all the information received is recorded, 0 none of it
B   spatial frequency of lines on test phantom
C   product
D   100%, by definition

5.11   C E
B   used in treatment planning but not simulation
C   other scintillation crystals are bismuth germanate and cadmum tungstate
D   contrast resolution decreases at higher spatial resolution

5.12   A D
B   decreases
C   increases area radiated
D   beam hardening
E   usually increased

5.13 A B C D

B   narrow window width

E   but scatter corrections can be made

5.14 B C D E

A   the crystal loses its piezoelectric properties at this temperature. (350°C for lead zirconate titanate)

B   resulting in vibration and the production of ultrasound waves

C   this reduces the 'ring down' time (expressed as the Q factor) and therefore gives the crystal more time in the receiving mode

E   because of D

5.15 B D

A   reduced at focus

B   registration error

D   Rayleigh-Tyndall scatter increases at frequency[4]

E   e.g. with cysts, indicates good image quality

5.16 B C E

B   other checks include a grey scale test, resolution test, frame rate, measurement accuracy and sensitivity

5.17 A C E

B   caused by static field

D   increases it

E   for hydrogen nuclei there only two spin orientations (I=1/2)

5.18 D E

A   gradient field

B   during RF pulse only

C   increasing slope decreases slice thickness

5.19 B

A   22 hours

B   generators usually changed weekly

C   saline

D   high grade alumina (Al_2O_3)

E   lead shielded and frequently desk mounted

5.20 A C D E

A   sensitivity 0.1%

B   no change

D   in absence of attenuating material

5.21 A B E

A all laryngeal cartilages may normally calcify except epiglottis and corniculate (elastic cartilage)
C remains open to 15 years of age
D adult 9-22 mm, child 5-14 mm

5.22 A B C D

B usually pontine branch but may arise from AICA
C branches at the geniculate ganglion
E 1 cm

5.23 B E

A do not meet
C asterion
E (strictly between them.) Persists into adulthood in approximately 10%

5.24 B C D

D the right drains the superior saggittal sinus, the left the straight

5.25 A B C D

A the caecum may be 9 cm in diameter
B jejunum up to 3.5 cm, ileum up to 2.5 cm
E always pathological

5.26 C D E

A T12
B pedicle of T12
C common iliac arteries and median sacral artery

5.27 D E

A L5
B only the right suprarenal vein
C right
D left enters the left renal vein

5.28 A E

B costocervical trunk
C 1st part of axillary artery
D 2nd part of axillary artery, with lateral thoracic. From 3rd part arise subscapular and two circumflex humeral branches

5.29 B

A C6
B it supplies upper 1/3, left gastric lower 1/3, and aortic branches middle 1/3
C 25 cm
D to the left
E anterior

5.30 A E

A but also increases in frequency with age
B 15 cm
D not true rings

5.31 A B E

A hence waist fracture leading to avascular necrosis of the proximal portion of the bone
C 2nd, 3rd and 4th
D pisiform appears at 10 years

5.32 A B C

A 1st bone to ossify (in membrane beginning in 5th week of fetal life)
B in order, next hamate, triquetral, lunate, trapezium, scaphoid, trapezoid and pisiform
D appears at 6 years
E appears at 3 years

5.33 C E

A end artery
D supplies the thumb

5.34 A D E

B superficial femoral vein
C joins the anterior tibial vein and enters the popliteal vein

5.35 A D

B penile, bulbous, membranous and prostatic
C prostatic portion
D distally dilated to form navicular fossa
E 20 cm

5.36 A B C

A the remnant of the urachus
D lateral wall
E piriformis

5.37   **A B**
   C   is lateral to the vein
   D   cords and branches
   E   teres major, where it becomes the brachial artery

5.38   **A B**
   C   8
   D   bilateral
   E   three roots

5.39   **A B C D**
   C   and inferior surface
   D   7 mm on ultrasound, 10 mm on radiographs
   E   no ligament supports the gallbladder

5.40   **A B C**
   B   lamina papyracea
   D   inferior floor
   E   inferior floor

5.41   **A D**
   B   radiologist
   C   mandatory
   D   right upper quadrant pain, especially in an obstructed system
   E   urograffin 150

5.42   **A B C E**
   A   maximum intrathecal dose 3000 mg
   C   in order to look for cerebellar tonsillar descent
   D   prone. The needle is not advanced after CSF is encountered, whereas it may in lumbar approach
   E   and any other patients who may be taking phenothiazines

5.43   **C**
   B   the cephalic vein should be avoided if possible because its acute angle of entry into the axillary vein inhibits the flow of contrast media
   D   simultaneous bilateral injections avoid flow artefact
   E   separate injections, otherwise an unobstructed side will preferentially fill

5.44   C D
   A it is much more expensive
   B 0.5-0.75 mg IV, 1-2 mg IM
   C it is a protein. Although this side effect is not just limited to those with peptic ulceration
   D antagonizes insulin
   E is contraindicated in suspected phaeochromocytoma, insulinoma

5.45   A B
   C water soluble contrast until it is established that there is no possibility of contaminating the peritoneum
   D the balloon should be gently inflated to secure it near the opening of the track
   E continuous screening to prevent obscuring detail by further injection of contrast media

5.46   A D E
   B 1:1,600
   C 40%
   D Ansell recommends prednisilone 50 mg orally 13, 7 and 1 hour before administration plus chlorpheniramine 4 mg and ephedrine 15-30 mg both given 1 hour before administration but the role of steroids is still unclear

5.47   A C D
   B decreases
   C shortens T_1 therefore can reduce TR

5.48   A
   B medial malleolus
   C middle of the plantar aspect of the foot
   D on the apex of the patella
   E 5 cm above the upper border of the symphysis pubis

5.49   B C D
   E tube angulation is required to clearly demonstrate the zygomatic arches

5.50   A C E
   A this is the most commonly used radiopharmaceutical in renal studies
   B ^{123}I Hippuran
   C also useful for demonstrating renal morphology
   D used to the size shape and position of the kidneys and therefore demonstrate scarring and cortical thinning

5.51   **A E**

   A   but has the disadvantage of not being organified in the follicles and giving a high background count

   B   it is cyclotron produced and has a shortish half-life (13.6 h)

   C   it gives a high thyroid and total body radiation dose

   D   parallel hole collimator

   E   may block uptake into gland

5.52   **A C E**

   B   useful with extrinsic compression to demonstrate anatomical relationships

   D   LPO

5.53   **D**

   A   extending

   B   flexing, prevents passage into the trachea

   C   inserted at this time

   D   air collects in the antrum and duodenal cap facilitating the tube's passage

   E   water can be infused but nothing should be swallowed because the patients pharynx has been anaesthetized

5.54   **A B D E**

   A   also to show the level and nature of a large bowel obstruction

   B   also suspected perforation and carcinoma in ulcerative colitis

   C   skip lesions maybe obscured by faecal residue

   D   to exclude perforation and toxic megacolon

   E   less abdominal discomfort following the examination

5.55   **C D E**

   A   1500 msec. In gradient echo a long TR would be about 100 msec

   B   30 msec. In gradient echo a short TE would be 5-10 msec

   E   proton density image. In gradient echo proton density has a short TE, small flip angle and a fairly short TR

5.56   **A B C**

   B   lipiodol is 0.5-2.0 ml per side

   D   the lower canaliculus. However, it is usual to perform bilateral simultaneous injections

   E   no more than 4 mm

5.57   **C D**

   A   33.3%

   B   right ventricle

   E   left atrium

5.58 C D E
   A this is only required if an opacity is seen on initial fluoroscopy
   B a higher iodine content (e.g. 290 or 350 mg iodine/ml) is needed
   C but it does not have to be completely removed
   D so that small uterine filling defects are demonstrated
   E alteratively, glucagon or inhaled amylnitrite

5.59 A B C D
   A methylglucamine salts cause a greater osmotic diuresis and therefore
       dilute the contrast medium in the collecting system
   B RCR recommendation
   C more slowly in the elderly
   D as long as there is no sign of cardiopulmonary disease
   E the converse is true

5.60 A B C D E
   C older children are seen to curl their toes when the bladder is full
   D this is especially important in boys so that posterior urethral valves are
       not missed
   E in order that any contrast that has refluxed and been missed during
       fluoroscopy is detected

BIBLIOGRAPHY

Armstrong, S.J., *Lecture Notes on the Physics of Radiology*, Clinical Press, Bristol, 1990.

Bell, G. and Finlay, D., *Basic Radiographic Positioning and Anatomy,* Balliere Tindall, London, 1986.

Chapman, S. and Nakielny, R., *A Guide to Radiological Procedures* (third edition), Balliere Tindall, London, 1993.

Curry, S.T., Dowdey, J.E. and Murry, R.C., *Christensens Physics of Diagnostic Radiology* (fourth edition), Lea and Ferbiger, Philadelphia, 1990.

Dendy, P.P. and Heaton, B., *Physics for Radiologists,* Blackwell Scientific Publications, Oxford, 1987.

Ellis, H. Logan, B. and Dixon, A., *Human Cross Sectional Anatomy Atlas of Body Sections and C.T. Images*, Butterworth-Heinemann, Oxford, 1991.

Ganong, W.S., *Review of Medical Physiology* (17th edition), Appleton and Lange, Norwalk, 1995.

Grainger, R.G. and Allison, D.G. ed., *Diagnostic Radiology* (second edition), Churchill-Livingstone, Edinburgh, 1992.

Gray, H. and Williams, P., *Gray's Anatomy* (38th edition), Churchill-Livingstone, Edinburgh, 1995.

Hornsby, V.P.L and Winter, R.K., *Aids to Part 1 FRCR,* Churchill-Livingstone, Edinburgh, 1988.

Keats, T.E., *Atlas of Normal Roentgen Variants That May Simulate Disease* (fifth edition), Year Book Medical Publishers, New York, 1991.

Lumley, J.S.P., Craven, J.L. and Aitken, J.T., *Essential Anatomy* (fourth edition), Churchill-Livingstone, Edinburgh, 1987.

McMinn, R.M.H., *Last's Anatomy* (ninth edition), Churchill-Livingstone, Edinburgh, 1994.

McMinn, R.M.H. and Hutchings, R.T., *A Colour Atlas of Human Anatomy*, Wolfe, London, 1977.

Plaut, S., *Radiation Protection in the X-Ray Department,* Butterworth-Heinemann, Oxford, 1993.

Royal College of Radiologists, *Making the Best Use of a Department of Clinical Radiology* (third edition), London, 1995.

Sharp, P.F., Gemmel, H.G. and Smith, F.W. eds., *Practical Nuclear Medicine*, IRL Press at Oxford University Press, Oxford, 1989.

Sutton, D. ed., *A Textbook of Radiology and Imaging* (fourth edition), Churchill-Livingstone, Edinburgh, 1993.

Weir, J. and Abrahams, P.H., *An Imaging Atlas of Human Anatomy,* Wolfe, London, 1992.

Whitehouse, G.H. and Worthington, B.S. eds., *Techniques in Diagnostic Imaging* (second edition), Blackwell Scientific Publications, Oxford, 1990.